Medicinal Plants of Barbados

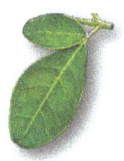

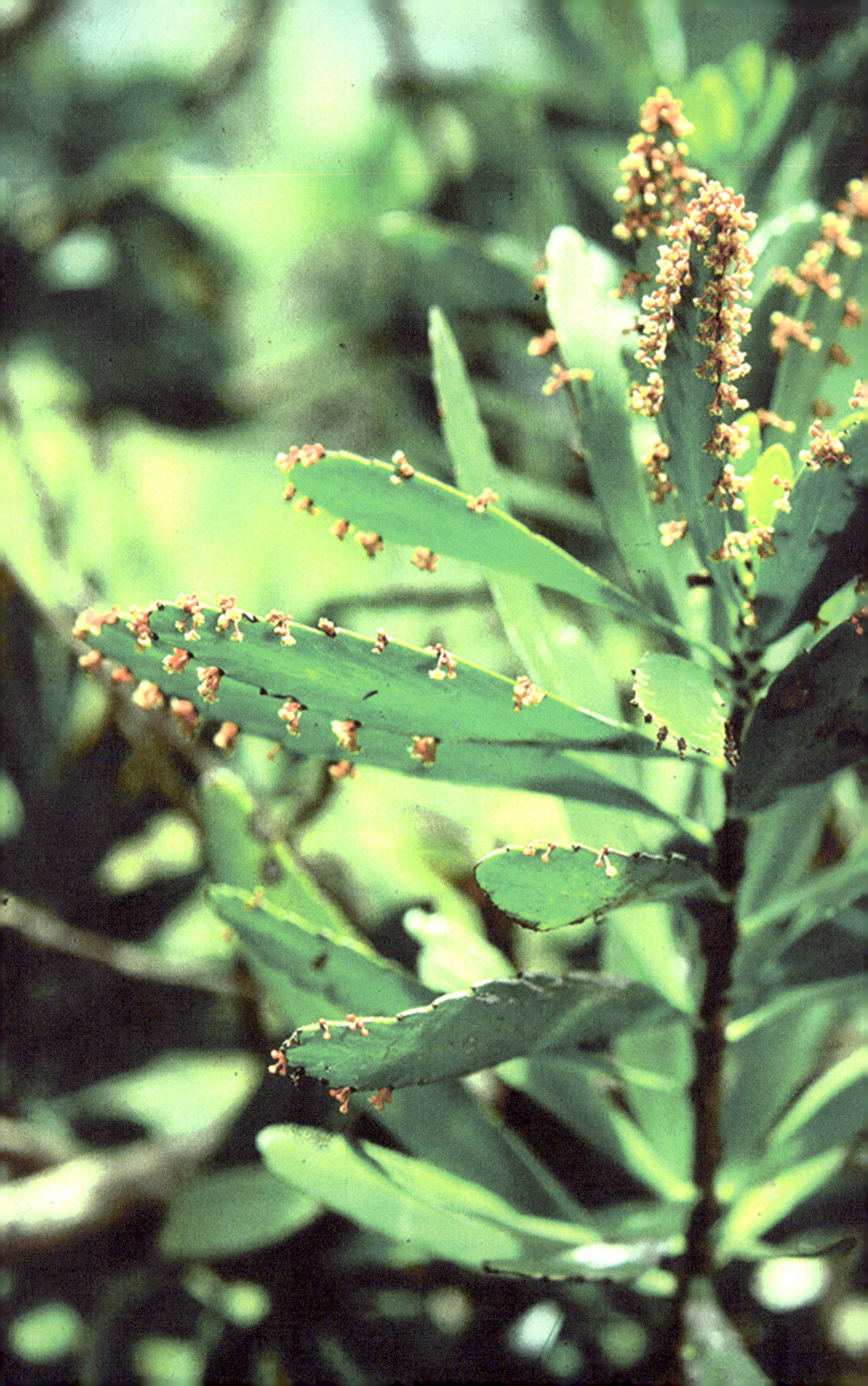

Medicinal Plants of Barbados

for the Treatment of Communicable and Non-Communicable Diseases

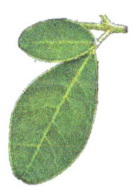

SECOND EDITION

DAMIAN H. COHALL

The University of the West Indies Press
Mona • St Augustine • Cave Hill • Global • Five Islands

The University of the West Indies Press
7A Gibraltar Hall Road, Mona
Kingston 7, Jamaica
www.uwipress.com

© 2026 by Damian H. Cohall

All rights reserved. Published 2026

First edition 2014

Second edition 2026

A catalogue record of this book is available from the National Library of Jamaica.

ISBN: 978-976-640-965-4 [pbk]
978-976-640-966-1 [EPub]

Cover and book design by Robert Harris
Set in PT Serif 10.5/15 x 27
Printed in the United States of America

Contents

Preface / **vii**

Acknowledgements / **ix**

1 **Treatment with Medicinal Herbs in Barbados** / **1**

Barbados – Discovery to its Geopolitical Landscape / **1**

Plant Biodiversity in Barbados / **8**

The Use of Plants as Medicines / **9**

The Evolution of Medicinal Plant Practices in Barbados / **15**

Factors Influencing the Use of Medicinal Plants in Barbados / **17**

2 **Traditional and Currently Used Medicinal Plants in Barbados for Communicable and Non-communicable Diseases** / **23**

Barbadian Medicinal Plants Used in the Treatment of Non-Communicable Diseases / **26**

   Cancer / **26**

   General Cardiovascular Diseases / **29**

   Diabetes / **30**

   Hypertension / **34**

   Neurodegenerative Disease / **49**

Barbadian Medicinal Plants Used in the Treatment of Communicable Diseases / **50**

   Bacterial Infections – Skin/Topical Ailments / **50**

   Bacterial Infections – Respiratory Ailments / **63**

CONTENTS

    Viral Infections – Cold, Influenza & Chicken Pox Virus / **69**

    Fungal Infections / **85**

Barbadian Medicinal Plants Used in Treatment Other than Communicable and Non-Communicable Diseases / **89**

    GIT Ailments / **89**

    Other Conditions / **94**

3   **Plant Nomenclature, Chemistry and Appraisal of Practices in Barbados** / **126**

    Plant Nomenclature / **126**

    The Chemical Profiling of the Medicinal Plants / **127**

    Appraisal of the Reported Bioactivity / **130**

    Best Practices Using Plant Based Medicines / **136**

4   **Development of Medicinal Plants into Drugs and Medicines** / **143**

    Drug Development Pipeline / **143**

    Cannabis: Prohibitive Shifts and the Development of a Medicinal Cannabis Industry / **148**

    Considerations / **156**

Glossary of Terms / **159**

Bibliography / **163**

Index / **173**

Preface

THIS WORK FOLLOWS THE FIRST EDITION OF *Medicinal Plants of Barbados for the Treatment of Communicable and Non-communicable Diseases* published in 2014. This edition provides an update on the historical and current knowledge and practices of the use of medicinal plants in Barbados. It also provides an updated list of medicinal plants used in Barbados, scientific appraisals of the plants' medicinal uses by an investigation of their bioactive constituents as well as pharmacological assessments of the practices. Barbados continues to have a strong base in the practice of botanical medicines. Consistent with the rest of the Caribbean region, the practice is criticised due to the lack of awareness of the developing data on the efficacy and safety testing of these plants. This book identifies common medicinal plants used historically and currently in Barbados for the treatment of common communicable and non-communicable diseases with laboratory and preclinical scientific assessments to support their uses.

Throughout the last decade, the scientific exploration of medicinal plants has become topical with the legislative reform for Medicinal Cannabis in Barbados, other Caribbean jurisdictions and globally. The scientific exploration of Cannabis for medicinal purposes has shown a value chain approach for investigating other medicinal plants which are more accessible than Cannabis. This edition will outline a practical guide towards harvesting and exploring the scientific value of medicinal compounds from plants used for medicinal purposes in Barbados.

The text starts by describing Barbados, its demographics and essential services from pre-independence to post-independence, which may have impacted the traditional practices of the inhabitants. It progresses into a comprehensive list of botanical medicines in Barbados which are primarily grouped based on their use to treat communicable and non-communicable diseases, and other miscellaneous ailments. The plants were grouped based on their taxonomical classification.

PREFACE

The chemical profiles of the plants were compared to established drug compounds, currently approved for the conventional treatment of illnesses, and to established phytochemicals. The book has approximately 157 entries of uses of medicinal plants. Approximately 92% of these entries identified for the treatment of communicable and non-communicable diseases in the review contain pharmacologically active phytochemicals, while 93% of the entries had bioactivities consistent with their reported use. These findings confirm the developing body of information to support the scientific basis of local botanical medicine. They also highlight a positive shift in the scientific investigations to support the practices from the publication of the first edition of *Medicinal Plants of Barbados,* which showed that 51% of the medicinal plant entries identified chemical compound(s) that have been associated with medicinal activity.

Medicinal Plants of Barbados (2nd Edition) has some other interesting highlights. It delves into a broader appraisal of the uses of the plants for medicines, which include the nomenclature and chemical profiling of medicinal plants, appraisal of the reported bioactivities and best practices using plants as medicines. Lastly, it highlights the prospects of the development of these botanical medicines into viable drugs and 'westernised' medicines through the drug development pipeline. It highlights the fledgling medicinal Cannabis industry and the opportunity for it to act as a catalyst for the development of medicinal plants into prescribable medicine.

The primary readers of this book are Barbadians and other Caribbean nationals who practice the use of herbal remedies and are keen on validating their uses. The secondary audiences are academics who wish to investigate these herbal remedies as sources of new drug compounds and clinicians who wish to be guided about bioactivities of the plants and possible drug-herb interactions. The book presents insightful information to both groups about the possible uses of herbal remedies. This book is by no means advocating the irrational use of any medication but is a resource to facilitate retention and possible use of traditional treatment approaches with plants to benefit society.

Acknowledgements

I EXTEND MY GRATITUDE TO Professor Sean Carrington, Professor Emeritus of Botany, Faculty of Science and Technology at the University of the West Indies, Cave Hill. Professor Carrington approved the use of his photographs in this publication. His work, which led to the publication, *Wild Plants of Barbados*, was instrumental in identifying the common names and some uses of the medicinal plants. He also assisted in the verification of the scientific names of the plants and ensured that they were consistent with the most recent advancements in phylogeny.

I extend my gratitude to my co-authors of two key scientific manuscripts on medicinal plants in Barbados that were published in the *West Indian Medical Journal (West Indian Medical Journal* 2012; 61 [1]: 17–27) and *Frontiers in Pharmacology (Frontiers in Pharmacology* 2021; 2021; 12: 713855) respectively. I also wish to acknowledge my other co-authors who worked collaboratively in conceptualizing, planning, and execution of other studies cited in the book. Contributions of photographs from Mr. Jacques Fourrnet and Father Mark de Silva are greatly appreciated. The kind collaboration of the Land and Survey Department in Barbados for the map of Barbados outlining parishes and major towns is also acknowledged. Lastly, I must acknowledge the efforts of Ms. Tatijana Vujicic for her exemplary efforts in the research and compilation of some of the data which contributed to this edition of the book.

This work is dedicated to my family, especially my wife, Tamecia Cohall and my mom, Deita Hamilton, who continue to inspire my fortitude. Finally, I thank God for his wonderful creation and the ability that He has bestowed upon me to study his marvellous works.

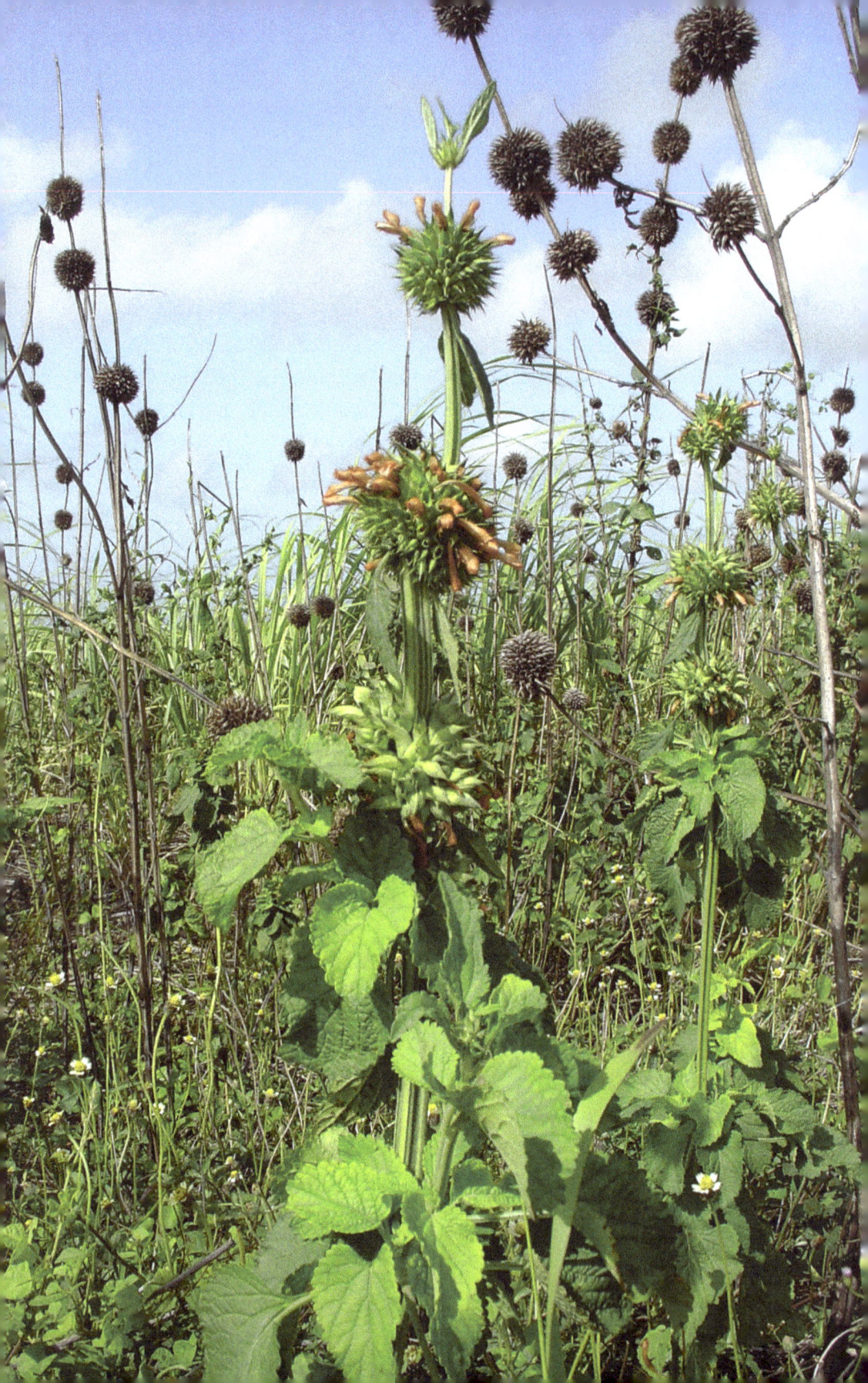

1

Treatment with Medicinal Herbs in Barbados

BARBADOS – DISCOVERY TO ITS GEOPOLITICAL LANDSCAPE

Barbados is an island in the Lesser Antilles of the West Indies with a land mass equal to 166 square miles. It is the most south-eastern island of the Caribbean Archipelago and records of its first encounter by Europeans dates as early as the sixteenth century, by the Portuguese after the discovery of other Caribbean territories in the Greater and Lesser Antilles. Its name derived from the *Los Barbudos* which symbolically identifies the island as the *Bearded Island* from the vast number of Bearded fig-trees (*Ficus citrifolia* Mill.) (1). The island was uninhabited upon its initial encounter by Europeans but historical notes highlight that it was visited by Amerindian settlers from neighbouring territories for food and other natural resources (1). It became a British colony between the seventeenth and twentieth centuries and remained under colonial rule throughout the transatlantic slave trade until its independence in 1966 (2).

Barbados was a part of the West Indian Federation during 1958–62. The West Indian Federation was established by The British Caribbean Federation Act 1956 which formed a multinational governance structure for its members (3). Post-Independence, the constitution of 1966 allowed for the formation of a governance structure which was similar to the British parliamentary system. The head of state remained the British

MEDICINAL PLANTS OF BARBADOS

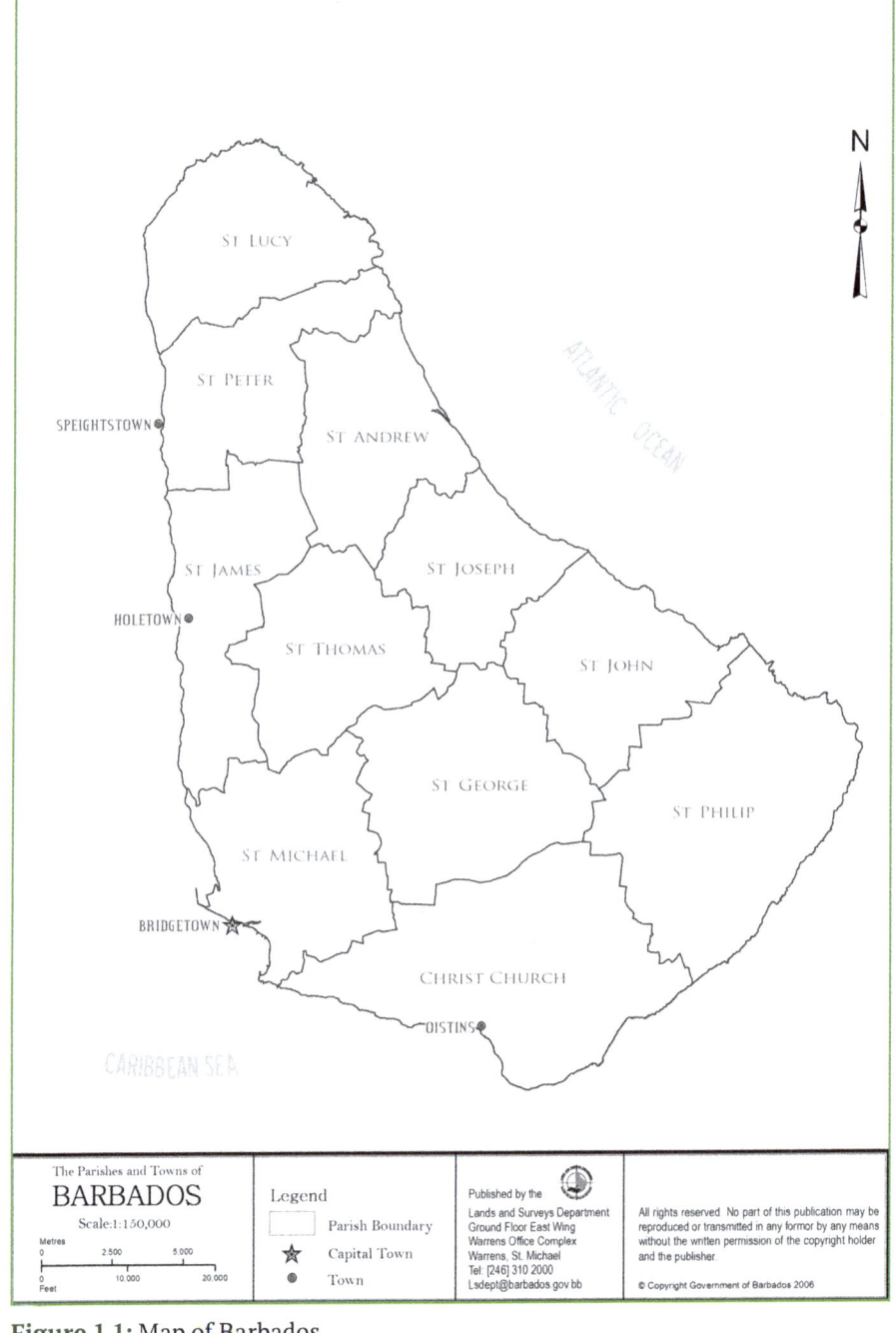

Figure 1.1: Map of Barbados

monarchy and was represented by a governor-general until 2021 (4). The island has two main political parties which were established by the trade and labour movements, the Barbados Labour Party, and the Democratic Labour Party. With the failed West Indian Federation in the 1960s, the Caribbean heads of states of Barbados, Guyana, Jamaica, and Trinidad and Tobago formed the Caribbean Community (CARICOM) in 1973 to facilitate functional cooperation while still maintaining their sovereignty. Today, CARICOM is a grouping of twenty countries: fifteen Member States and five Associate Members. Prior to CARICOM, there was the Caribbean Free Trade Association (CARIFTA) in 1965. Barbados has been a member of CARIFTA and CARICOM from their inception (5). In 2021, Barbados relinquished its colonial ties with Britain and transitioned into a republic state.

Population Demographics and Cultural Landscape

Barbados has a population of approximately 269,090 with an urban population of 31.2% in the 2021 census (4). Tourism is the main income earner for the country and according to the Barbados Statistical Service, stay-over tourist arrivals for 2023 and 2024 were 636,603 and 704,340 respectively(6). The median age of the population is 42.5 and the sex ratio is 1:1.07 males to females. The main ethnic groups in Barbados are people of African descent (or mixed between African and European descent) at approximately 92.4% and unmixed European descendants at 2.7% followed by an even smaller number of inhabitants who originated from the Middle Eastern and Indian subcontinents (4,7). Unlike Trinidad, Guyana and Jamaica, there was no settlement of indentured Asian labourers during the quests for constant and cheap labour during 1838–1917 after the abolishment of slavery (2). There is also an expatriate community mainly from Britain and North America, which completes the population (4). According to Government of Barbados, the 2021 official census indicated that 75.6% of the population is Christian (7). The demography of the Christian faith based on magnitude in descending order was Anglican (13%), Pentecostal (19.5%), and Seventh Day Adventists (5.9%). The Methodists (11%) and Roman Catholics

(1.9%) are considered as significant minority groups. The non-christian religious group represents 16.8% of the population and includes Rastafarians, Muslims, Hindus, Jews, and Baha faith members (4).

Socioeconomics of the Island

Prior to the COVID-19 pandemic, Barbados was ranked 58th among other countries globally based on its human development index in 2019. Three important factors contributing to this index is the country's social services (including its education system), health care and social welfare. According to the UNDP's Human Development Report 2020, data culminating in 2019 revealed that i) the expected years of schooling was 15.4, ii) the island's literacy rate among persons aged 15 and older was 99.6% and iii) the literacy rate of persons aged 25 and older with at least secondary education was 93.2% (8). These indices are enabled by a government-funded primary and secondary school system which is free for attendees. Also, there are facilities for technical and vocational education, a community college and a teachers' college. The island has one of the five main campuses of The University of the West Indies. The tuition of Barbadians who matriculate to the University are funded by the government (4). Health is explored in more detail later in chapter 1. The life expectancy at birth was reported at 74.3 and 77.7 years for males and females respectively in 2019 and the health expenditure was 6.8% of the gross domestic product for the same period (9). Other important human development indices in UNDP's 2020 report outlined a low poverty rate of 2.5%, an employment to population ratio of 58.5% for ages 15 and older and a low homicide rate of 9.8 per 100,000, up to 2019 (8).

Communicable and Non-communicable Diseases in Barbados

Diseases are broadly classified as communicable and non-communicable diseases. These broad categories describe the aetiology of the diseases. Communicable diseases are infectious conditions which are transmissible by air, vector, host, and sexual transmission. Non-communicable diseases are non-transmissible and non-infectious as the name suggests. These may also be considered chronic conditions which are classified as degenerative/progressive. These include conditions such as cancer, respiratory and cardiovascular diseases, autoimmune and nutritional based disorders. Overall, these two sets of conditions contribute significantly to epidemiological data on mortality and life expectancy, two indicators adjudicating the health of populations.

According to data from the World Health Organization's (WHO) Global Health Observatory Data Repository in 2019 prior to the pandemic, Barbados's life expectancy at birth (males/females) was 74.3/77.7 years and probability of dying between the age of 15 and 60 years for males/females (per 1,000 population) was 129/74 (9). These data suggest that the health and well-being of Barbadians was among the highest compared to its fellow Caribbean member states at that time. According to a United Nations Economic Commission for Latin America and the Caribbean (ECLAC) report in 2011, Barbados's life expectancy at birth ranked among the top five territories in the Caribbean and ECLAC member states for both sexes, during the period, 1950 to 2050 (10).

Historically, the enslaved population, Amerindians and Europeans were afflicted with similar ailments (11). The coast of West Africa, the common site of the embarking of slaves to vessels en route to the Caribbean, was considered a breeding ground for infectious diseases. The plethora of communicable diseases, more so than the non-communicable ones increased during the transport across the middle passage (11). The enslaved Africans were more resilient to these conditions than their counterparts. Their resilience may have been linked to acquired immunity due to exposure to similar tropical diseases along the coast of West Africa, genetic predisposition, and their familiarity with various healing methods for these conditions. A recent study was able to identify genetic differences between Europeans and Africans which influences immune responses to bacterial and viral pathogens (12). Reports from large case-control studies conducted in East and West Africa indicated genetic polymorphisms which contribute to innate immunity against malaria. These studies provide strong evidence that the most common African Glucose-6-Phosphate

Dehydrogenase (G6PD) deficiency variant, G6PD A–, is associated with a significant reduction in the risk of severe malaria for both G6PD female heterozygotes and male hemizygotes (13). Nevertheless, the communicable/infectious diseases which were noteworthy in Barbados during the seventeenth to nineteenth century are:

1. Smallpox
2. Chicken pox, measles, whooping cough and mumps
3. Diphtheria
4. Sore throats
5. Colds, influenza, and croup
6. Pneumonia and tuberculosis
7. Leprosy, yaws
8. Sexually transmitted diseases
9. Topical infections
10. Diarrhoea
11. Typhoid
12. Tetanus and neonatal tetanus
13. Yellow fever and malaria
14. Filariasis
15. Scabies, lice
16. Parasitic worm infections

During the same period, the noteworthy non-communicable diseases in Barbados were nutritional based and conditions resulting from trauma as shown below:

1. Protein energy malnutrition: Kwashiorkor and Marasmus
2. Vitamin deficiencies: Pellagra and Beriberi
3. Lead poisoning, alcoholism and traumas

It is widely accepted that the nutritional-based conditions may have affected children more so than adults. During the same period, it is hypothesized that natural selective forces across the transatlantic channel: diet, environmental-genetic factors, trauma and psychological factors along with the more recent increase in sedentary lifestyles may have led to the increase in cardiovascular diseases and other chronic non-communicable diseases in the Caribbean and territories in the Americas. A comparative study of hypertension in persons of African descent by Cooper et al. (1996) was able to demonstrate a gradient in the prevalence of hypertension among seven populations of West African origin from Nigeria through the Caribbean to Maywood, Chicago in the United States of America (14). Barbados recorded the highest prevalence of hypertension among the Caribbean territories in the study and has been noted as a potential study site to further investigate hypotheses focusing on the development of multifactorial diseases, especially cardiovascular conditions in the western world. The establishment of the national Chronic Non-communicable Disease Registry by the Ministry of Health in 2008 has supported that effort.

Health data in Barbados have indicated an age-standardized mortality rate of 436.7 (per 100,000 population) in 2016 (9). This mortality rate adjusts for differences in the age distribution of the population by applying the observed age-specific mortality rates for each population to a standard population. When the major contributors of the standardised figures are accessed based on disease categories, chronic non-communicable diseases account for a significant majority of the overall figure (9). This indicates either better public health strategies to mitigate communicable diseases inclusive of the use of antibiotics and vaccines or chronic non-communicable diseases being the highest contributor of mortality rates due to the adoption of western lifestyles. The 2015 Health of the Nation study in Barbados found that 1 in 10 adults has a non-communicable disease (NCD). Eighty per cent of men and 90% of women have at least one risk factor, and one-third of adults are being managed for at least 1 NCD (15). The most common risk factors for NCDs in Barbados include high blood pressure, high fasting plasma glucose, high cholesterol and high body mass-index (16). The age-standardised mortality rate per 100,000 for NCDs increased from 749.19 in 2013, to 912.34 in 2019 (16). The age-standardised mortality rates by cause (ages 30–70 years, per 100,000 population) for the following non-communicable diseases in 2016 were: cancer – 732, diabetes mellitus – 286, cardiovascular diseases – 947 and chronic respiratory conditions (inclusive of asthma and obstructive pulmonary disease) – 114 (9). In 2019, Chronic NCDs contributed to 8 of 10 top causes of death in Barbados. These included:

1. Ischaemic Heart Disease – conditions related to the imbalance of the heart's oxygen demand and the supply of oxygen to the heart
2. Stroke
3. Diabetes
4. Prostate cancer
5. Chronic Kidney Disease
6. Colorectal cancer
7. Breast cancer
8. Hypertensive related heart disease

The major communicable diseases affecting Barbadians and the people of the Caribbean are sexually transmitted diseases, tuberculosis, cholera, dengue, zika, chikungunya, malaria, influenza and most recently, the SAR-COV-2 (9, 17, 18). The prevalence of HIV among Barbadian adults aged 15 to 49 years was 0.8% in 2019. The mortality rate of tuberculosis, excluding the tuberculosis associated with HIV, was 9 per 10,000 of the population in 2019 (9). The case fatality rate for SAR-COV-2 virus among males and females in Barbados were reported to be 0.39% and 0.25% during 2020–2021 (19). In 2019, prior to the SAR-COV-2 pandemic, only one communicable disease was ranked in the top 10 causes of death related to morbidity and this was lower respiratory tract infection (9).

The total expenditure on health as a percentage of the gross domestic product was approximately 6.8% in 2019. This figure is comparable with figures among the other English-speaking countries in the Caribbean.

PLANT BIODIVERSITY IN BARBADOS

Globally, plants are classified according to shared physical characteristics and based on morphological characteristics alone, some 300 such groups have been recognised as plant families. However, the application of molecular approaches to phylogeny is resulting in major taxonomic revisions and the recognition today of some five hundred families (20). Within each family, there may be several genera and species. A species may have several varieties which are the single botanical taxon of the lowest rank (21). Note that the taxonomical order starts with the Plantae kingdom but filters to the plant species and its varieties.

Barbados' vegetation is strongly influenced by the seasonal tropical climate associated with the island's geographical location, which supports the rich diversity of plants. In the days of early colonisation by the Europeans, there were thousands of plant species on the island, However, in more recent times there are only about 600–700 species of plants that can be found in the wild, two of which are considered endemic to the island (22, 23). The reasons for the decline in plant species will be discussed later in Chapter 1.

Similar to other works, such as *Medicinal Plants of the West Indies* by Edward S. Ayensu and Caribbean-based plant electronic repositories such as TRAMIL – Program of Applied Research to Popular Medicine in the Caribbean, in this book, different plant species in Barbados which are known to have medicinal properties are identified and placed within their respective plant families (24, 25). This book is an updated version of its first edition, which probes deeper than the physical classification of the medicinal plants in Barbados. It summarises the known medicinal plants' chemical and pharmacological characteristics that can be used to explain their possible uses in traditional medicine. Particular attention will be directed to plants used by Barbadians for treatment of infectious communicable diseases and chronic non-communicable diseases.

THE USE OF PLANTS AS MEDICINES

Medicinal plants have been considered as the cornerstone for the development and evolution of medicines from as early as 3000 BCE (26). Since then, plants and other elements of nature have been sources of drugs and the study of this sub-division of pharmacology is called pharmacognosy. The study of materials used by ethnic and cultural groups as medicines is called ethnopharmacology. These established areas within the discipline of pharmacology have led to the development of highly recognised herbal remedies in their natural or commodified forms, and pharmaceuticals from lead compounds identified from the plants.

Compounds isolated from plants with discrete bioactivities towards animal biochemistry and metabolism are termed phytochemicals; and many conventional drugs have their beginnings from these phytochemicals. The phytochemical group of alkaloids is a remarkable example of plant compounds contributing to the development of conventional drugs both as derivatives and in their original extracted forms. Drugs such as morphine, quinine, atropine, and vincristine are all alkaloids derived from plants. Other phytochemicals of interest are flavonoids, phenolic acids, terpenoids, esters, phytosterols and saponins. Phytochemistry will be explored in greater detail in Chapter 3.

The Historical Context of the Use of Medicinal Plants

Plants have been used a source of medicine since 3000 BC. The earliest artefact of this therapeutic practice was discovered on a Sumerian clay slab dating back to that period. Details of its discovery highlighted the first medicinal plant formulary with over 250 plant species with methods of preparation for their medicinal uses (27). In some instances, the use of these herbs was described as magical as the biological effects were incomprehensible. In the fifteenth century, apothecaries were developed, and these were the first retail entities in which herbal preparations could be sourced in ancient European territories. During the nineteenth and twentieth centuries, the development of the natural and biomedical sciences contributed to the understanding of the biological and medicinal effects of plants. These sciences also contributed to the development of the pharmaceutical industry in which a significant number of plant derived compounds were evaluated and became active pharmaceutical ingredients (26).

Traditional medicine is deeply rooted across various cultures and its practice is strongly informed by religious, spiritual and societal norms of our ancestors (28). Documented practices of the ancient origins of herbal medicine includes the Traditional Chinese Medicine, Traditional Indian Medicine (otherwise called Ayurveda) and the European approaches (27, 29, 30). However, African practices and lesser-known ethno-practices by other cultures fail to be highlighted among documented traditional practices as they tend to be oral without written folk recipes. While most cultures have retained the core values and morals of their ancestral heritage over time, the use of traditional medicine by the African diaspora has undergone continuous transformation, knowledge 'seepage' and reinvention in concert with the socio-political issues related to its acceptability in countries outside of the continent where Africans were taken or migrated (28). Societies have adapted to keep pace with the ever-evolving world and the attitudes, knowledge, and practices of generations of people. These changes are primarily influenced by local domestic issues and globalisation, and have demonstrated the malleability of cultural practices as civilisations cross pollinate and evolve (31).

The Origins of Medicinal Plants in the Caribbean

The cultural practices of the Caribbean inclusive of the use of medicinal plants emanated from the convergence of ethnic practices of various ancestral peoples influenced by global knowledge (28). While some practices are well preserved from their initial ancestral traditions, others have morphed to accommodate varying ideologies. One must recall that Caribbean society comprised of the descendants of indigenous people (Arawak and Carib mainly), West Africans, European colonisers, and the indentured servants. The ancient origins of their cultural practises informed the use of plants in the Caribbean and added significantly to the region's biocultural diversity.

Ancestral Belief Systems and Influences in the Caribbean

The Caribbean is a striking example of a region whose culture and traditions were continually influenced by a gradual evolution of practices in accordance with external interactions and pressures that came with an increasingly globalised world. The evolution of cultures and traditions started with waves of the Amerindians influx into the Caribbean. It then continued from the sixteenth century by means of European colonisation of the region, the transatlantic slave trade and the emigration of Asian indentured labourers (2, 28). As a result, traditional medicine in the Caribbean, inclusive of the use of plants, is a convergence of the practices of the indigenous people, emigrants, and enslaved West Africans.

Amerindian, European and West African Healing Traditions and Other Traditions

The Caribbean islands were inhabited mainly by the Amerindians inclusive of the Arawaks and the Caribs prior to European colonisation. The belief system of the Amerindians was based heavily on a spiritual understanding whereby good and bad spirits were affiliated with well-being. Bad spirits were typically considered to be affiliated with misfortunes and illness, hence treatment approaches were holistic and the plants transcended the physical benefits to promote emotional, spiritual and community well-being (32). Tobacco was used by healers or Shamans to facilitate communication with the spiritual realm to guide diagnosis and patient care. Pineapple and Arrowroot were used for urinary and digestive ailments, sores, and other lesions. The use of these two plants became a prime example of cultural exchange during colonisation as these plant-based therapies became a part of European pharmacopeia (33).

A similar holistic approach to healing was practised in West Africa. This was described as tripartite and included herbalism, spirituality, and divination. The West African belief system identified a divine power who is a healer and manifested this healing through plants, spirits, and deities with the assistance of healers or Shamans on earth. Health and well-being which not only focused on the proper functioning of the body, mind and spirit but also on the quality of relationships with ancestors were important factors contributing to health (34). Any imbalance in these factors contributing to health was identified as an illness and were considered to originate from evil or malevolent spirits, neglected ancestors, witchcraft or sorcery or physical causes. The diagnosis and treatment of illness includes consultation with the spiritual world and remedies were spiritual and/or herbal depending on the nature of the illness (34).

The medicinal system in Europe around the time of colonisation of the Caribbean was based on the humoral theory of health and disease. The body was considered to be composed of four humours inclusive of yellow and black bile, blood, and phlegm. Each of these humours was aligned with specific determinants of health and disease. Yellow bile was associated with hot and dry, black bile was associated with cold and dry, blood was associated with hot and moist, and phlegm was associated with cold and moist. Both the imbalances and the quality of the humours were related to the nature of the illnesses. For example, yellow bile caused illnesses with increases in body temperature (hyperthermia) and black bile caused conditions with low body temperature (hypothermia). Imbalances resulted from improper regulation of the six "non-naturals" inclusive of i) air, ii) food and drink, iii) motion and rest, iv) evacuations and retentions, v) wake and sleep and v) passion and emotion. Treatment within the European medicinal practice was to restore balances of the humours, hence hot diseases were treated with cold remedies and vice versa (35).

Indentured labourers immigrated to the Caribbean during the nineteenth and twentieth centuries to supplement the workforce after the abolishment of slavery. They were primarily of Chinese and East Indian origins. The Chinese traditional medicinal practice is based on the Yin-Yang concept which suggests that the universe is composed of two opposites (Yin and Yang). The balance of these two paradigms is required for health and well-being and is related to illness. Medicinal plants are used in Chinese traditional medicine to balance Yin and Yang and were classified into four energies: hot and warm (associated with Yin) and cold and cool (associated with Yang). The use of plants such as Ginseng, Ginger and Garlic, popular herbs in the Caribbean, had in 2500 BCE been documented in the book "Pen Tsao" with other plants used in ancient Chinese medicine (29). The East Indians would have practiced the holistic ancient Indian system of medicine, Ayurveda.

The basis of this practice is that the universe is made of five elements: i) air, ii) water, iii) space or ether, iv) earth and v) fire, which collectively form three humours of the human body called doshas. Similar to some of the practices described above, imbalances in the doshas resulted in illnesses. Ayurveda treatments included five mechanisms to detoxify the body which are based on the use of plants (30). The use of nutmeg, pepper and cloves in current Caribbean medicinal practices can be attributed to ancient Ayurvedic practices (27). Although indentured labourers did not contribute to the Barbados workforce in any significant way compared to other Caribbean territories, the cross-fertilisation of cultures across the Caribbean has impacted the cultural practices on the island.

Cultural Syncretism and Evolution of Healing Traditions

During the seventeenth to nineteenth centuries, the Europeans enslaved and transported approximately five million Africans to the Caribbean. The enslaved Africans were subjected to horrific living conditions which increased their risks of contracting non-communicable and communicable diseases. While the enslaved were seen as valuable commodity by the European settlers, their well-being was selectively prioritised based in their value. Due to the vast number of imported enslaved African compared to European settlers (inclusive of their medical practitioners) and the decimation of the Amerindians, the healing practices of the West and Central Africans became the predominant method of healing for the enslaved (28). These practices were vital to survival in the Caribbean islands due to the plethora of tropical infectious diseases which originated in the Caribbean, Europe and also from the coast in West Africa (11). European colonisers observed the medicinal practices of the indigenous and African healers and would bring this knowledge and practice back to Europe without acknowledging the indigenous people and Africans in the process. The Europeans divorced the cultural components of the healing practices when documenting their observations, thus isolating the plants and their associated physical therapeutic properties (35). Some of these adopted and adapted practices became mainstay European medicinal traditional practices as described above. Also, the European colonisers grew to distrust African healers as they believed the healers embodied African culture and thus could inspire hope and resilience amongst the slaves. This was seen as a threat to the economic model of slavery which required the slaves to be stripped of their heritage and remain vulnerable. A lot of cultural aspects of the medicinal practices were suppressed and there was forced indoctrination of Eurocentric values, attitudes, and religious beliefs. This syncretism between African and European cultures led to Neo-African practices and religious movements such as Vodou, Santeria, Shango and the Spiritual Baptists. Spirituality and supernatural beliefs are evident in healing practices associated with these Afro-Caribbean religious movements as well as the European and the Chinese "hot-cold" premise for the use of herbs (28).

THE EVOLUTION OF MEDICINAL PLANT PRACTICES IN BARBADOS

The use of medicinal plants in Barbados evolved along the historical influences observed in the rest of the Caribbean but without significant cultural input from indentured servants. Cultural syncretism and the suppression of African cultural practices influenced cultural habits and the use of traditional medicine among the slaves and subsequent generations. This suppression of culture was more evident in the smaller islands with smaller plantations and fewer slaves. The lack of arable uncultivated lands and opportunities on the islands post-emancipation led to the freed slaves working as labourers on plantations and this perpetuated the values and constructs of slavery even after its abolishment in 1834. This was more evident on the smaller islands in the Caribbean such as Barbados (36). For example, in the 1800s, Barbados enacted its first anti-Obeah laws, directed against persons who practiced the 'magical or supernatural' charm or power to promote the insurrection or rebellion of slaves. This in practice, would have also suppressed healers who were using herbs to heal. Variation of these laws continued for two centuries (37). The Anglican church served the planter hierarchy in Barbados and was involved in the deculturization of Africans by dismantling tribes and discouraging social gatherings (38). The cultural axis of African traditions inclusive of the use of medicinal plants was suppressed by these deliberate actions by the state and church. Therefore, the local pharmacopeia of traditional healing traditions which developed during this time was not confined to one group's knowledge and practices, but was instead the retained knowledge and uses of the plants culminating from the deculturalization and cultural convergence during the time of colonisation (39).

Despite the deculturalization and suppression of African heritage and practices, the use of medicinal plants has remained an important aspect of modern Barbadian culture. A study by Cohall et al. (2011) investigated the factors influencing the use of herbal remedies by Christians in Barbados. The study was conducted in ten Anglican churches and one Moravian church (40). It indicated that at least 33.6% of the respondents used herbal remedies to treat different conditions including chronic diseases. Approximately 58% of the users of herbal medicines are women, and this is possibly due to their maternal and nurturing functions within the family unit. The findings on the use of herbal remedies in this study were also corroborated with the findings of Dr Sonia Peter's work on Medicinal and Cooling Teas of Barbados in *African Ethnobotany in the Americas* which identified similar percentages of Barbadians using herbal remedies in the wider society (41). A study by Vujicic and Cohall (2021) outlined that 75% of residents in a rural district in Barbados use medicinal plants (42). This supports the rural-urban divide on the retention of indigenous and ancestral practices. Other ethnopharmacological studies in Jamaica and Trinidad and Tobago reported prevalence of use of herbal remedies of 60% and above but some of these study populations may not be generalisable to national populations (43, 44). According to the World Health Organization, in 2011 between 70% and 95% of the world population used botanical preparations for medicinal purposes and 80% or more use plants for some part of primary healthcare (45, 46). Global, regional and rural percentages of use of plants for medicinal purposes are higher than urban trends in Barbados which could be a direct result of deculturalisation during and after the time of slavery among other factors.

FACTORS INFLUENCING THE USE OF MEDICINAL PLANTS IN BARBADOS

Iris Bayley, a Barbadian horticulturalist, has suggested that while herbal medication may not be as popular as it was in the past, it is still quite regularly used by the Barbadian population (23). The following factors that influenced the prevalence of use of medicinal plants post emancipation can be considered.

Ancestral Influences

The ancestral influence on the current practice of medicinal plants has been documented earlier in this chapter. The types of diseases which impacted the inhabitants of the island over the sixteenth to twentieth centuries and the treatment methods have informed current practices (11, 23, 39). Most of the uses of medicinal plants locally are for infectious communicable conditions which were more prevalent during the period of slavery. The naming of the herbal treatments, for example, cooling teas, aligns with ancestral belief systems and cultural syncretism between Eurocentric and Afrocentric healing practices mentioned earlier in the chapter. These practices are criticised as being non-scientific, but this critique fails to highlight the 'uncontrolled' indigenous scientific methodology (including random observations in nature, over several generations and locations) used by our ancestors in making their inferences on efficacy and safety of these herbal remedies. This are contrasted to randomised 'controlled' clinical trials considered to be the gold standard for assessing efficacy and safety of conventional pharmaceutical products.

The ageing and rural populations of the island are tied tied closer to the ancestors' practices and they are the ones who tend to use medicinal plants more frequently (40–42). However, there are concerns that these ancestral practices are being lost due to lack of permeation of knowledge and practices to the younger generations.

Education

Educational advancement represented an opportunity for freed slaves to escape the trauma and indignation of enslavement, and the rigors of plantation labour. It allowed the African population of Barbados to develop an identity rooted in literacy and education to counter the inherent racism and social biases of a colonial society. Prior to independence, the education system was under British colonial rule and significantly influenced the deculturalization of the former enslaved Africans. It also safeguarded the economic interest of the colonisers by indoctrinating the former enslaved Africans to accept their societal role as subservient God-fearing labourers. Thus, education played a significant role historically in dismantling the traditional healing beliefs as well as other African practices. Many Afro-Barbadians adopted western medicine and Christianity, and traditional African practices were largely confined to the uneducated Afro-population (38). There has been an enhancement in education opportunities on the island post-independence, which has further distanced locals from traditional practices and created more scepticism of the benefits of herbal remedies. Studies from other Caribbean territories with similar educational systems have shown that the use of herbal remedies is inversely proportional to the level of education attainment; the use of medicinal plants was consistently lowest among persons with tertiary education and highest among persons with low education attainment (47–49). Interestingly, some educated individuals are keen to use commodified medicinal plants whose traditional uses are scientifically validated (50). In addition, most of the currently available systematic reviews address herbal preparations which are marketed and widely used in industrialised countries. However, some herbs, especially indigenous species, used in Caribbean traditional medicine seem to be less investigated (51). Most Barbadian herbal remedies have yet to be subjected to the same rigorous efficacy and safety trials as prescription drugs. Furthermore, since conventional medicines have also been demonstrated to be very effective, Barbadians may not feel the need to use alternative medications.

Universal Health Care

The 1969 Health Services Act of Barbados, Cap. 44 and the Drug Services Act 1980 provide the framework which ensures that Barbadians receive universal healthcare coverage and access to quality drugs at affordable prices regardless of their socio-economic circumstances (52, 53). There is a fee for the use of laboratory equipment, X-ray machines, a specific category of drugs and drug services. Public healthcare is provided in the polyclinics and in the Queen Elizabeth Hospital, which is the only public general hospital in Barbados. In 2023, there were approximately 677 doctors, 1,035 nurses and 367 pharmacists in the public health sector for which expenditure incurred by government was US$175.5 million (54). There are no established provisions for the administration of traditional medicine within the public health sector.

The Benefit Service Scheme provides free drugs to patients 65 years and older, and to patients aged 16 years and younger, leaving patients between the ages of 16 and 65 years to purchase some drugs at their own expense. The drugs that are free to the age gap (16–65 years) are limited to those used to treat only certain disorders, such as diabetes, hypertension, cancer, asthma and epilepsy (55). While it may be postulated that health insurance, access to universal health care and affluence may reduce the population's need to use traditional healing practices, studies in 2011 and 2021 varied on the association of health insurance and the use of herbal remedies with a positive association in the latter study (40, 42). This difference in outcomes in the two studies may be due to the difference in study populations with the former being a cross-sectional sample of Barbados and the latter being a sample from rural Barbados. Secondarily, there is difference in opinion on the use of plant-based remedies in the twenty-first century. Herbal products are not only accessible in raw forms but also as commodified products which are in demand to a wide demography of persons who aim to live healthier lifestyles with greater emphasis on disease prevention (56). Also, information about the use of herbal remedies is also widely available. It is postulated that persons within the age categories supported fully under the Benefit Drug Scheme, (16 and younger and 65 years and older), may use less plant-based medicines to treat conditions. The same was considered for persons within the 16–65 age group supported by the scheme for specific conditions who may use plant-based medicine for conditions not supported by the scheme. No firm associations were able to be drawn based on the data presented in the studies mentioned above.

Employment Status, Income and Sociocultural Factors

Studies in other Caribbean territories, Jamaica and Trinidad and Tobago, suggest that persons who are employed are more likely to buy over-the-counter (OTC) medicine than use medicinal plants for aliments and that the use of herbal remedies is more prevalent among persons in the lower income bracket (50, 57). Additionally, income was also associated with the type of herbal remedies used by persons. While persons in the lower income bracket preferred native and traditional herbal remedies, those in a higher income bracket were keen on using herbs of European and North American origin or commodified products (50). No significant associations between employment, income and use of medicinal plants have been reported in Barbados to date.

A large proportion of the slave population relocated from rural to urban communities after the abolishment of slavery with the hope of improving their job prospects and quality of life. A major part of this shift was not only physical but sociocultural, to conform to the Eurocentric culture of the colonial upper class which was more predominant in the urbanised areas. Some of these practices included subscribing to the Catholic and Protestant churches, visiting western-trained physicians, and receiving a western-influenced education. On the contrary, Afro-Barbadians who remained in the rural areas retained a stronger cultural identity associated with their African heritage (28, 42). This observation still holds in modern society as studies have shown that the use of herbal remedies is higher among persons in rural areas (42, 49, 57). The ageing population, who reside mainly in remote areas of the island, is tied closer to the immigrants' practices and they are the ones who tend to use herbal remedies predominantly (40, 41). These practices have been passed down to younger generations for continuity.

There is also a general belief that that herbal remedies are safer than westernised health care systems and medicines. This prompts people to self-diagnose and treat their ailments with herbal remedies. Even the most sophisticated of the local population will do this (23). Some of the local patient population reported that the patient-physician relationship influenced their attitudes towards accessing traditional medicine. Physicians were focused on the pathophysiology of the disease, diagnosis and then treatment without taking a holistic approach towards the care of the patient (58, 59). The perception exists that this approach is a perpetuation of colonial healing practices in contrast to the holistic traditional practices of the ancestors.

Religion

Religious movements have been an important aspect of the cultural impression of the pre- and post-colonial landscape in Barbados. While syncretism between African and European cultures led to various Afrocentric religious movements such as Vodou, Santeria, Orisha and the Spiritual Baptists in some Caribbean territories, the religious landscape in Barbados has remained primarily influenced by the Eurocentric Christian religious movement (7, 28). The 2021 official census indicated that 75.6% of the population is Christian. The denominations of the Christian faith are primarily Anglican (13%), Pentecostal (19.5%), Seventh Day Adventists (5.9%), Methodists (11%) and Roman Catholics (1.9%). Christianity has the common belief that plants were created to be used as food and for the healing of the nation. The Bible, the book of faith used by Christians, has several references about this:

1 Kings 21:2, "And Ahab spake unto Naboth, saying – Give me thy vineyard, that I may have it for a garden of herbs, because it is near unto my house: and I will give . . .".

1 Kings 4:33, "And he spake of trees, from the cedar tree that is in

Lebanon even unto the hyssop that springeth out of the wall: he spake also of beasts, and of fowl, and of creeping things, and of fishes";

A more specific reference to medicinal herbs is found in the books of John and in Revelations:

John 19: 29, "Now there was set a vessel full of vinegar: and they filled a sponge with vinegar, and put it upon hyssop, and put it to his mouth";

Revelations 22:2, "the leaves of the trees are for healing of the nation"; and Psalms 51:7,"Purge me with hyssop, and I shall be clean: wash me, and I shall be whiter than snow".

The non-Christian religions comprised 16.8% and includes Rastafarians, Muslims, Hindus, Jews, and Baha faith members (7). These have practices which includes the use of plant materials as religious sacraments and for healing. Of this minority group, Rastafari which originated in Jamaica in the 1920s and was introduced to Barbados in 1975, is the most strident in its religious right and freedom on the use of *Cannabis sativa* as its sacrament and also for its medicinal value (60).

Deforestation and Land Development

There has been a decrease in the number of species of plants including those with known medicinal properties in Barbados. In the days of colonisation, there were thousands of plant species; however, there are only about 600–700 species of plants in the twenty-first century, both imported and indigenous (22, 23). The reduction in the number of plant species on the island in the pre-colonial era was due to deforestation to make room for sugarcane plantations and other vegetable crops (23, 41). In the post-colonial era, land was cleared for the development of urban centres and residential lots on the coasts of the island. More recent residential developments have been more inland which can further impact the number of plant species available on the island (61). Fortunately, the island maintains some of its natural plant diversity in natural gullies like Welchman Hall Gully, and developed reserves and gardens like the Andromeda Botanic Garden. These areas remain untapped for agricultural and housing developments in Barbados and retain some of the island's plant species in their natural habitat.

2

Traditional and Currently Used Medicinal Plants in Barbados for Communicable and Non-communicable Diseases

THIS CHAPTER PROVIDES A COMPREHENSIVE LIST of traditional medicinal plants, and their current uses or role as botanical medicines in Barbados. It builds on the repository of uses listed in the first edition of *Medicinal Plants of Barbados* by including current practices; some of which may not be easily categorised under the broad headings of communicable or non-communicable conditions. The main aims of this chapter are to i) demonstrate that the investigation of the phytochemical properties of these medicinal plants within their respective taxonomical groups can preliminarily validate some of the medicinal claims associated with the use of the plants and ii) to document studies on the plant extracts and the purified and characterised phytochemicals, inclusive of toxicological and efficacy studies, which can be used to substantiate the claims of the plants' medicinal uses.

The Barbadian medicinal plants are categorised in three main sections which are outlined based on traditional and current practices of treating communicable diseases, chronic non-communicable diseases and a miscellaneous category of ailments which may be related to the two former groups. These ailments were selected for the review based on the incidence and prevalence among the inhabitants of the island, historical and current. The infectious diseases considered for this review are mainly bacterial, viral infections (inclusive of the common cold, influenza and chicken pox) and fungal infections. The non-communicable diseases considered are cancer, hypertension and other cardiovascular related disorders and diabetes mellitus. The sections allow for the entry of information on the taxonomical classification, scientific and common names of the plants, the preparation of the plants, the bioactive compounds with the medicinal effects and literature sources supporting the use of the plant for the reported medicinal application. In some instances, the chemical profiles of the plants were compared to established drug compounds approved for the conventional treatment of illnesses and to established phytochemicals. The scientific nomenclature of all the plant families and species were verified using the Kew Medicinal Plant Name Services (MPNS) and the final list of plants was reviewed by a plant taxonomist for accuracy. Some plant entries have vouchered samples from ethnopharmacological studies which were submitted to the Herbarium at The University of the West Indies, Cave Hill Campus.

An extensive review of the literature was conducted mainly from PUBMED indexed journal articles to substantiate the medicinal claims cited later in the text. The information captures the limited but rich plant biodiversity of the island, local use of the plants and their identified phytochemical compounds. The data outlines approximately 157 entries of medicinal plant use. Approximately 92% of these plant entries identified for the treatment of communicable and non-communicable diseases in the review contain pharmacologically active phytochemicals, while 93% of the plant entries reported bioactivities consistent with their reported use. Nutritional chemical profiles were limited in this text while emphasis was placed on phytochemicals considered to be associated with the management of the specific ailments and diseases. The information shows the data collected from the investigations conducted on these plants. Most of these investigations are laboratory and animal-based investigations of the plant extracts or isolated compounds from the extracts. These data highlight that plants have specific bioactivities which support their use to treat illnesses/diseases in traditional medicine. While the data outline some alignment with the plants' uses, clinical significance must be demonstrated for the plant preparation to be considered an alternative to conventional approaches which have been standardised and have demonstrated efficacy and safety. Other uses of herbal remedies inclusive of complimentary and preventative approaches are less contentious.

BARBADIAN MEDICINAL PLANTS USED IN THE TREATMENT OF NON-COMMUNICABLE DISEASES

CANCER

Spondias mombin L.
Hog /Gully Plum
Family: Anacardiaceae
Local Preparation: Tea of the barks by hot infusion.
Bioactive Chemical Profile: Phenolic compounds (geraniin, galloyl geraniin), sterol and terpenoids (3-hydroxy-22-epoxystigmastane and stigmasta-9-en-3,6,7-triol) (1)
Pharmacological Activity: Hydro-ethanolic extract of *S. mombin* leaves showed significant antioxidant activity in an *in vitro* DPPH assay with radical scavenging activity ranging from 66% to 76%. (1)

Annona muricata L.
Soursop
Family: Annonaceae
Local Preparation: Leaves boiled for cancer prevention. Skin of fruit dried and ground into powder followed by extraction by decoction or infusion for breast cancer. (2, 3)
Bioactive Chemical Profile: Acetogenins, alkaloids and phenols. (4)
Pharmacological Activity: A variety of anti-cancer activities (anti-proliferative, apoptotic, anti-metastatic) have been verified against cell lines *in vitro*. (4, 5) These activities have been reported in a two-stage skin papillomagenesis model in mice, breast (MCF7, MDA and SKBR3), prostate, pancreatic, lung and colon (HCT116 and HT-29) cancer cell lines.

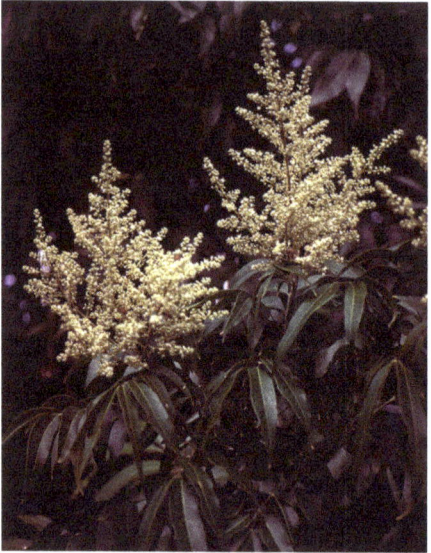

Hog /Gully Plum

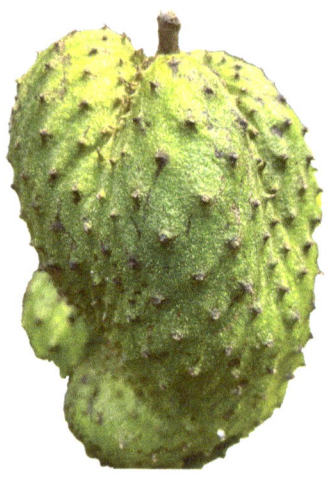

Soursop

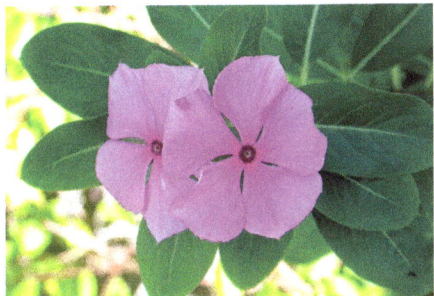
Madagascar Perwinkle

Catharanthus roseus (L.) Don [DC017]
Madagascar Perwinkle
Family: Apocynaceae
Local Preparation: Hot infusion of leaves and stems for anti-cancer properties.
Bioactive Chemical Profile: Monoterpene indole alkaloids, e.g. catharanthine, vindoline, vincristine and vinblastine. (6)
Pharmacological Activity: Vincristine & vinblastine are approved anticancer pharmaceutical compounds. (6)

Carica papaya L. [DC011]
Pawpaw, Papaya
Family: Caricaceae
Local Preparation: Root is boiled for colon cancer. (3)
Bioactive Chemical Profile: α-tocopherol, lycopene, flavonoids and benzylisothiocyanate. (7)
Pharmacological Activity: Antiproliferative, and growth inhibitory activities exhibited against various tumour cell lines. The medium polarity fraction of papaya leaf juice (0.03–0.003 mg/mL) showed potent growth inhibitory (IC_{50}=0.02–0.07mg/mL) and cytotoxic activities on prostate tumour cells after 72 hours of exposure to the cell lines. Also, an upregulation of immunomodulatory genes inclusive of CCL2, CCL7, CCL8 and SERPINB2 have been reported. (7, 8)

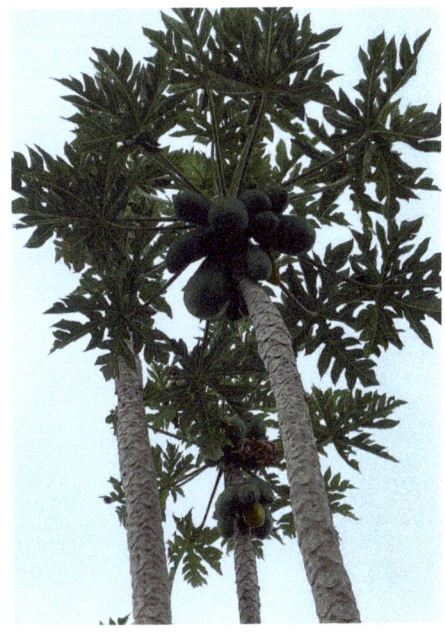
Pawpaw, Papaya

Phyllanthus amarus Schum.
Seed-under-Leaf
Family: Euphorbiacae
Local Preparation: Decoction of the leaves.
Bioactive Chemical Profile: Lignans, flavonoids, hydrolysable tannins (ellagitannins), polyphenols, triterpenes, sterols and alkaloids. (9)
Pharmacological Activity: Extracts inhibited breast (MCF-7) and lung (A549) carcinoma cell growth with IC_{50} values ranging from 50–180 μg/

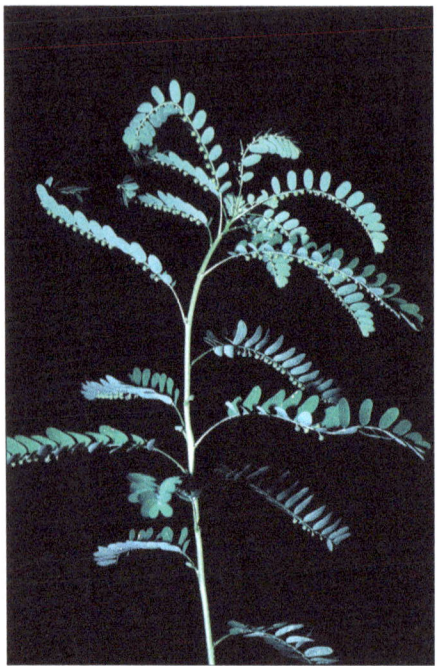
Seed-under-Leaf

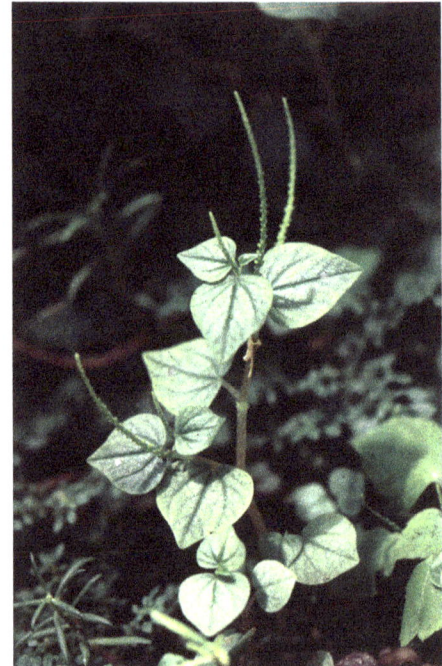
Shining Bush

ml and 65–470 µg/ml for methanolic and aqueous extracts respectively. Also, there was reduced cancer cell invasion and migration, adhesion of the cells, and induced apoptosis at concentrations ranging from 20–200 µg/ml for methanolic extracts and 50–500 µg/ml for aqueous extracts in similar cell lines. (10)

Peperomia pellucida (L.) Kunth
Shining Bush
Family: Piperaceae
Local Preparation: Hot infusion or decoction of the whole plant.
Bioactive Chemical Profile: Peperomin E; other phytochemicals in the methanolic extract. (11)

Pharmacological Activity: Cytotoxic activity against human epithelial kidney (HEK 293), human cervical cancer (HeLa) and human hepatic carcinoma (HePG2) cell lines. Peperomin E and another compound inhibited growth of promyelocytic leukemia (HL-60), breast cancer (MCF-7), and cervical cancer (HeLa) cells with IC_{50} values ranging between 1.4 and 9.1 µM and between 1.8 and 11.1 µM respectively. (11, 12)

Physalis angulata L.
Cow Pops, Poppers
Family: Solanaceae
Local Preparation: Hot infusion of the leaves.

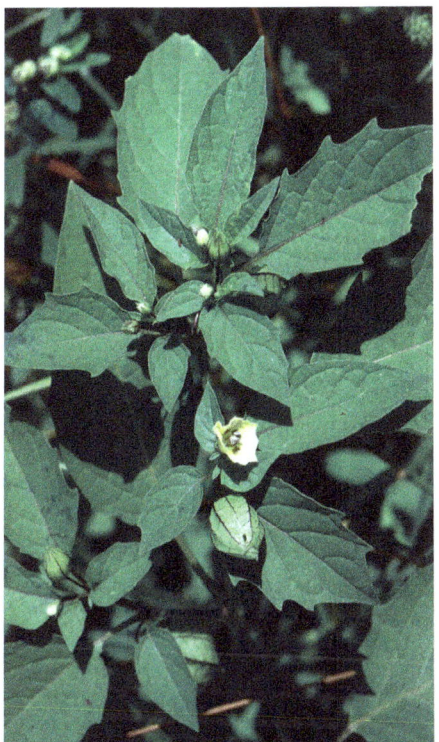

Cow Pops, Poppers

Bioactive Chemical Profile:
Phenolic compounds, e.g., flavonoids, withanolides and physalins. (13)
Pharmacological Activity: Ethyl acetate extracts at a concentration of 5–15 µg/mL significantly inhibited the migration and invasion of highly metastatic human tongue squamous carcinoma (HSC-3) cells in a wound-healing repair assay and trans-well assay. Other cellular effects also supports anti-metastatic, anti-proliferative, and cytotoxic activities in human umbilical vein endothelial cells (HUVECs) *in vitro*. (14, 15)

GENERAL CARDIOVASCULAR DISEASES

Calotropis procera (Aiton) Aiton f.
French Cotton
Family: Apocynaceae
Local Preparation: Decoction of various parts of the plant inclusive of the latex, leaves and bark.
Bioactive Chemical Profile:
Calotropin, calotropagenin, calotoxin, calactin, uscharin, amyrin, amyrin esters, uscharidin, coroglaucigenin, frugoside, corotoxigenin, calotropagenin and voruscharine. (16)
Pharmacological Activity: The latex extract obtained from the plant exhibits potent anti-inflammatory activity in various animal models that is comparable to standard anti-inflammatory drugs. The ethanolic extract *C. procera* latex at an oral dose of 300 mg/kg three times daily for 30 days significantly reduced enzymatic biomarkers for myocardial infarction in an isoproterenol (20 mg/100 g)-induced model in albino rats. (16, 17)

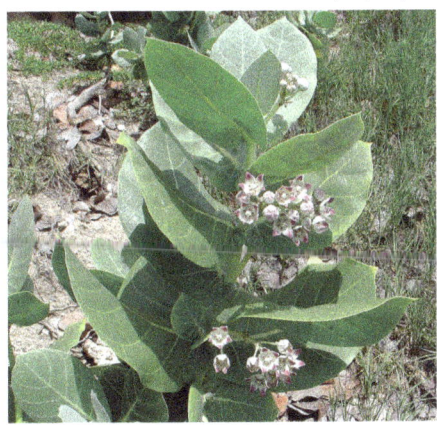

French Cotton

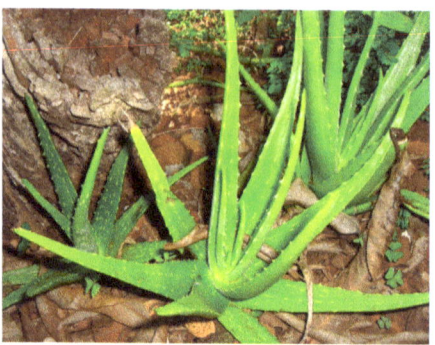
Aloe vera

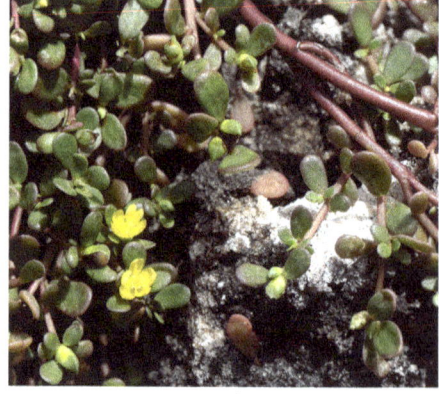
Pussley

Aloe vera (L.) Burm.f. [DC009]
Aloes
Family: Asphodelaceae
Local Preparation: Gel; ingested raw, blended with juice, decoction or infusion. (3)
Bioactive Chemical Profile:
α-tocopherol, carotenoids, ascorbic acid, catechin hydrate and caffeic acid. (18)
Pharmacological Activity: The aqueous extract of Aloe Vera gel administered daily at 30 mg/kg, interperitoneally significantly enhanced the bleeding time in mice and in combination with vitamin-K (10 mg/kg, interperitoneally) compared to control. (19, 20)

Portulaca oleracea L.
Pussley
Family: Portulacaceae
Local Preparation: Decoction of the plant.
Bioactive Chemical Profile:
Flavonoids, alkaloids (noradrenaline, dopamine & adenosine), fatty acids, terpenoids, polysaccharides, vitamins, sterols, proteins and minerals. (21)
Pharmacological Activity:
Alkaloids (noradrenaline, dopamine & adenosine) are cardio-active and sympathomimetic amines. Antioxidant, anti-inflammatory and antilipidemic activities of the plant extracts have also been reported. (21, 22)

DIABETES

Bidens pilosa L.
Duppy Needles, Monkey Needles, Spanish Needles
Family: Asteraceae
Local Preparation: Hot infusion of the leaves.
Bioactive Chemical Profile:
Flavonoids, polyacetylenic compounds (cytopiloyne) and tannins. (23)
Pharmacological Activity: Three polyacetylenic compounds of the plant reported glucose-lowering and insulin-

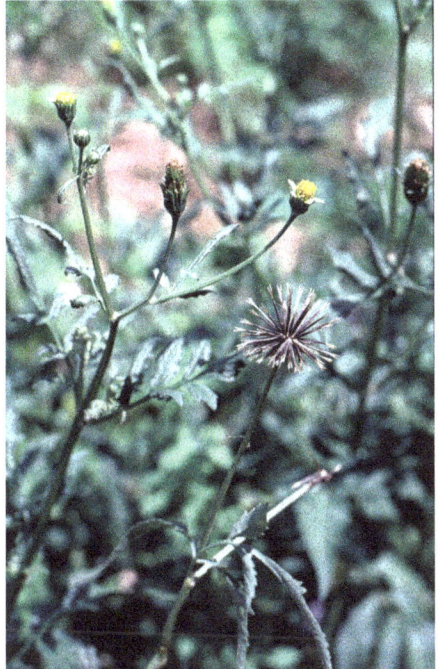

Duppy Needles, Monkey Needles, Spanish Needles

flavonoids, terpenoids, stearic acid, myristique acid and ellagic acid. (25)
Pharmacological Activity: In diabetic rats, single oral administration of the aqueous extract significantly reduced blood glucose levels by 75% and 58.22% respectively at a dose of 100mg/kg and 200mg/kg as compared to the initial blood glucose values. Antioxidant activities of the aqueous extract have also been reported. (25)

Tecoma stans (L.) Juss. ex Kunth
Christmas Hope, Elder Bush
Family: Bignoniaceae
Local Preparation: Hot infusion of the leaves.
Bioactive Chemical Profile: Rutin, β-sitosterol and alkaloids. (26, 27)
Pharmacological Activity: Studies have shown the ability of *T. stans* extracts to induce adipogenesis, improve glucose uptake, and decrease insulin resistance. (26, 27)

releasing activities in animal and human studies. Also, rats with Type 1 Diabetes mellitus treated with an aqueous extract of the leaves at a daily dose of 200 mg/kg orally for 4 weeks showed a better recovery of the glucose levels for two weeks compared to the control and other treatment groups. (23, 24)

Annona muricata L.
Soursop *(see entry on page 26)*
Family: Annonaceae
Local Preparation: Leaves dried and boiled.
Bioactive Chemical Profile: Alkaloids, tannins, coumarins,

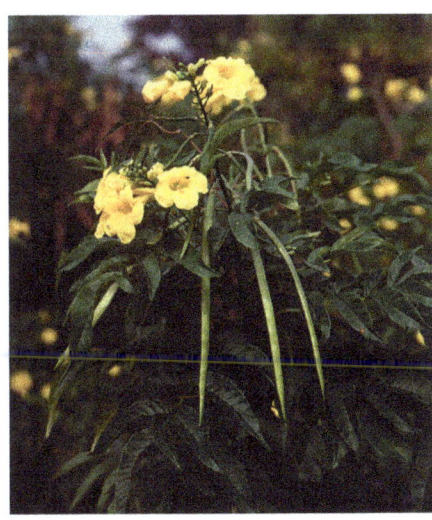

Christmas Hope, Elder Bush

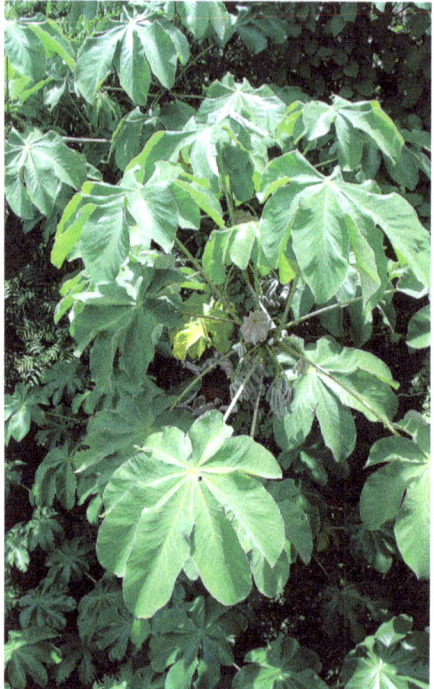
Trumpet Tree, Pop-a-Gun

Cecropia schreberiana Miq.
Trumpet Tree, Pop-a-Gun
Family: Cecropiaceae
Local Preparation: Hot infusion of the leaves.
Bioactive Chemical Profile:
Triterpenoids, flavonoids (flavone C-glycosides, flavonolignans and proanthocyanidins and chlorogenic acid. (28, 29)
Pharmacological Activity: Aqueous and methanolic extracts of the leaves belonging to other species of the genus Cecropia with chlorogenic acid showed a significant hypoglycemic effect upon oral administration in a streptozotocin induced diabetes mellitus rat model. (29)

Momordica charantia L. [DC002]
Cerasee, Miraculous Vine, Crapaud, Pumpkin, Lizard Food
Family: Cucurbitaceae
Local Preparation: Hot infusion of the dried leaves.
Bioactive Chemical Profile:
Proteins and peptides (momordins, momorcharins), terpenoids, saponins, flavonoids, phenolic compounds, essential oils and fatty acids. (30)
Pharmacological Activity:
Plant extracts showed a potential therapeutic benefit in diabetes and obesity related metabolic dysfunction in experimental animals and clinical studies. These effects are mediated by the possible induction of a lipid and fat metabolizing gene expression and by increasing the function of AMP-activated protein kinase (AMPK) and Peroxisome proliferator-activated receptor (PPARs). (30, 31)

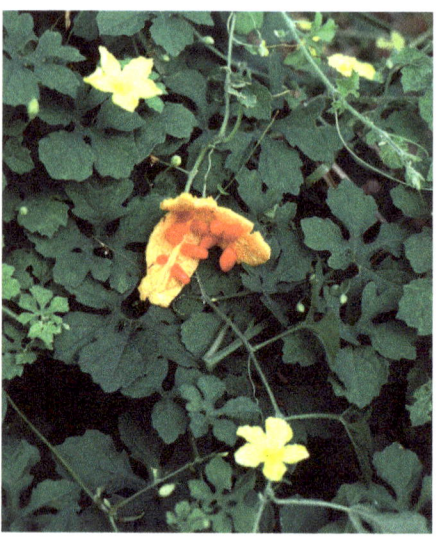
Cerasee, Miraculous Vine, Crapaud, Pumpkin, Lizard Food

MEDICINAL PLANTS IN BARBADOS FOR COMMUNICABLE AND NON-COMMUNICABLE DISEASES

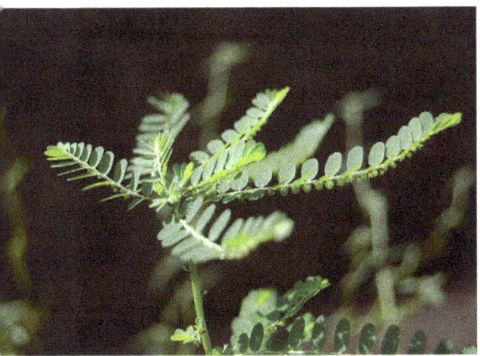

Seed-Under-Leaf

Phyllanthus niruri Linn.
Seed-Under-Leaf
Family: Euphorbiacae
Local Preparation: Infusion of the leaves and seeds.
Bioactive Chemical Profile:
Flavonoids (rutin, quercetin, quercitrin & astragalin), alkaloids, terpenoids, lignans, polyphenols, tannins, coumarins and saponins. (32)
Pharmacological Activity: Aqueous *P. niruri* extracts administered orally caused a reduction of blood glucose in an animal model and among diabetic patients. Also, the plant has flavonoid phytochemicals which have reported antioxidant and anti-inflammatory effects. (32, 33)

Azadirachta indica A.Juss.
Neem
Family: Meliaceae
Local Preparation: Hot infusion or decoction of the leaves. (2)
Bioactive Chemical Profile:
Nimbin, nimbidin, quercetin, limonoids, terpenoids, sterols, fatty acids, coumarins, azadiradione,

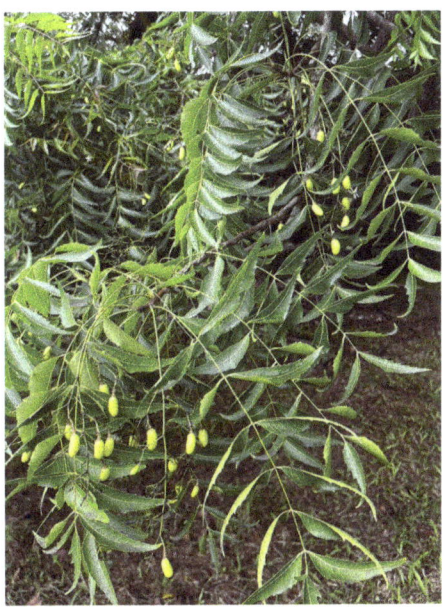

Neem

hydrocarbons, sulphur containing compounds and phenolics. (34, 35)
Pharmacological Activity: Plant extracts exhibited inhibitory activity against enzymes involved in diabetes and significant blood glucose-lowering effects. Also, the ethanolic extract of the *A. indica* leaves at an oral dose of 200 mg/kg normalized glucose level and lipid profile after streptozotocin induction of diabetes in rats. (36, 37)

Moringa oleifera Lam.
Moringa
Family: Moringaceae
Local Preparation: Hot infusion or decoction of the roots, leaves and stem. (2)
Bioactive Chemical Profile: Quercetin and kaempferol (38).

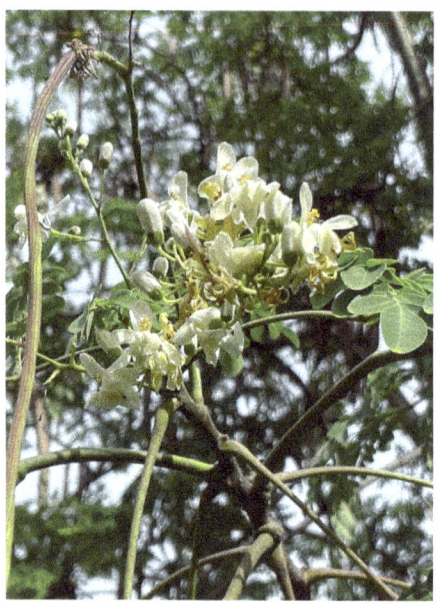
Moringa

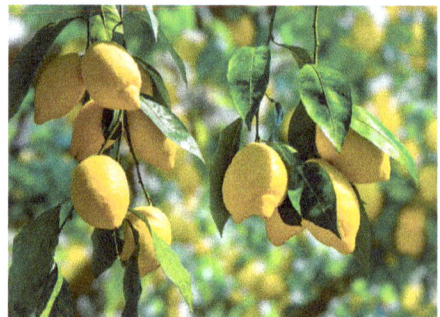
Lemon

Pharmacological Activity: Treatment with the methanolic *M. oleifera* extract at a daily dose of 150 and 300 mg/kg orally for 21 days reduced serum glucose levels, increased serum insulin levels, and reversed pancreatic islet cell damage in a diabetic rat model. (38)

Citrus limon (L.) Osbeck
Lemon
Family: Rutaceae
Local Preparation: Hot infusion of the lemon. (2)
Bioactive Chemical Profile: Flavonoids (hesperidin, rutin, nobiletin, naringenin, 8-prenylnaringenin, quercetin, diosmin and tangeretin). (39)
Pharmacological Activity: Aforementioned phytoconstituents have demonstrated potent anti-diabetic effects in a number of *in vitro* cellular cells (e.g., nobiletin and 3T3-L1 preadipocytes) and animal studies (e.g., 8-prenylnaringenin and C57Bl/6 mice). These flavonoids regulate biomarkers of glycemic control, lipid profiles, modulate signaling pathways related to glucose uptake and insulin sensitivity. (39)

HYPERTENSION

Justicia pectoralis Jacq.
Garden Balsam
Family: Acanthaceae
Local Preparation: Hot infusion or decoction of the leaves.
Bioactive Chemical Profile: Coumarins, flavonoids, steroids, triterpenoids and alkaloids. (40)
Pharmacological Activity: The hydroalcoholic extract (HAE) from the leaves of *J. pectoralis* have shown hypotensive related effects (anti-inflammatory, anti-oxidant and antispasmodic effects) in animals studies. (40)

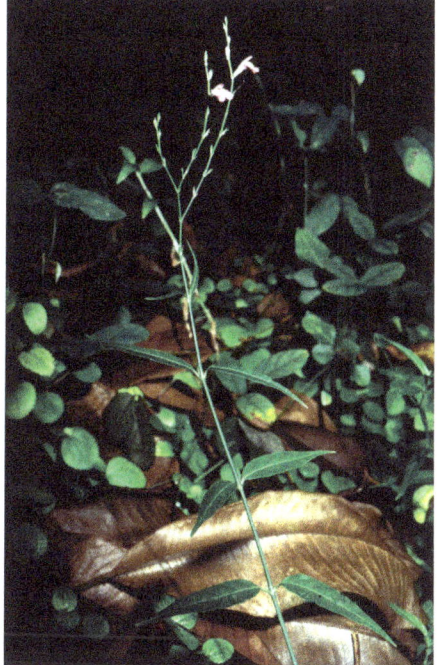
Garden Balsam

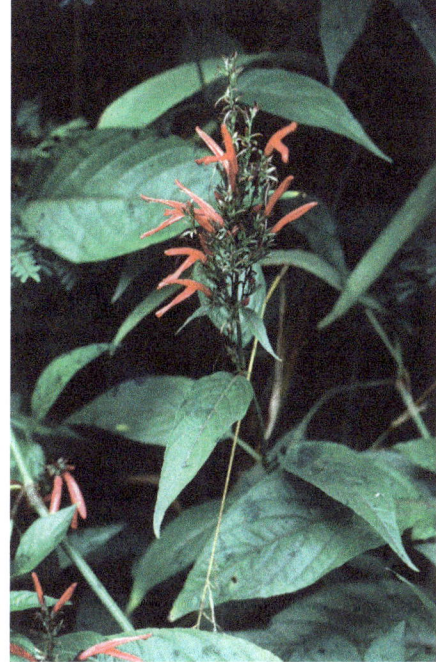
Bloodroot

Justicia secunda Vahl
Bloodroot
Family: Acanthaceae
Local Preparation: Hot infusion of the flowers and/or leaves.
Bioactive Chemical Profile: Flavonoids (esp. luteolin), tannins and anthocyanins. (41, 42)
Pharmacological Activity: An aqueous extract of the leaves of *J. secunda* at a dose of 5.55–55.55 mg/kg administered intravenously showed a potential antihypertensive effect on blood pressure of adrenaline induced hypertension in rabbits previously anesthetized with ethyl-urethane. (43)

Annona muricata L.
Soursop
Family: Annonaceae
Local Preparation: Leaves boiled then bottled and left in refrigerator overnight before drinking. (2)
Bioactive Chemical Profile: Phenolic compounds (e.g., cinnamic acid derivatives, p-coumaric acid) and reticuline. (44)
Pharmacological Activity: The effective concentration of the extracts causing 50% antioxidant activity, EC_{50} revealed that the pericarp and seed extracts had highest and least Angiotensin Converting Enzyme (ACE) inhibitory effects at 0.03mg/ml and 0.20 mg/ml respectively *in vitro* among

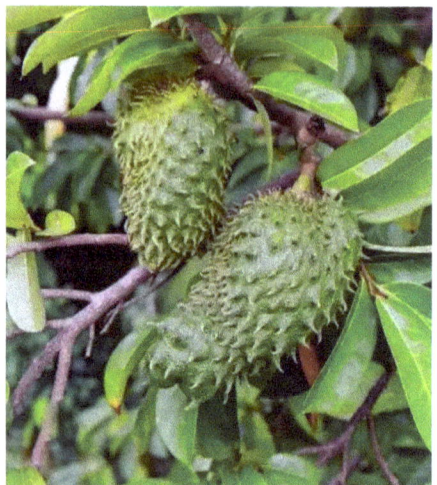

Soursop

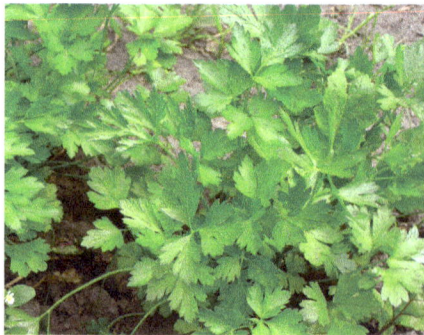

Parsley

other free radical scavenging effects. Also, an aqueous extract of *A. muricata* leaves at a dose of 9.17–48.5 mg/kg caused significant dose-dependent reduction in blood pressure without affecting the heart rates. (44, 45)

Petroselinum crispum (Mill.) Fuss
Parsley
Family: Apiaceae
Local Preparation: Hot infusion or decoction. (2)
Bioactive Chemical Profile: Apiin, 6"-acetylapiin, myristicin, apiol and coumarins. (46)
Pharmacological Activity: The aqueous extract of the aerial parts of *P. crispum* at an oral dose of 160 mg/kg daily for 7 days decreased the systolic, diastolic and mean arterial blood pressure in normotensive and hypertensive rats via a vasodilatory mechanism. (46)

Catharanthus roseus (L.) Don [DC017]
Madagascar Periwinkle
Family: Apocynaceae
Local Preparation: Decoction of the leaves.
Bioactive Chemical Profile: Monoterpene indole alkaloids, e.g. catharanthine, vindoline, vincristine, vinblastine and serpentine. (6)
Pharmacological Activity: Reserpine is an indole alkaloid and also an FDA approved antihypertensive agent (3); Serpentine is hypotensive. (6)

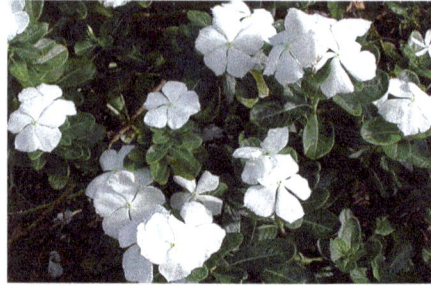

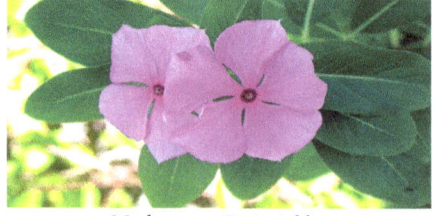

Madagascar Periwinkle

MEDICINAL PLANTS IN BARBADOS FOR COMMUNICABLE AND NON-COMMUNICABLE DISEASES

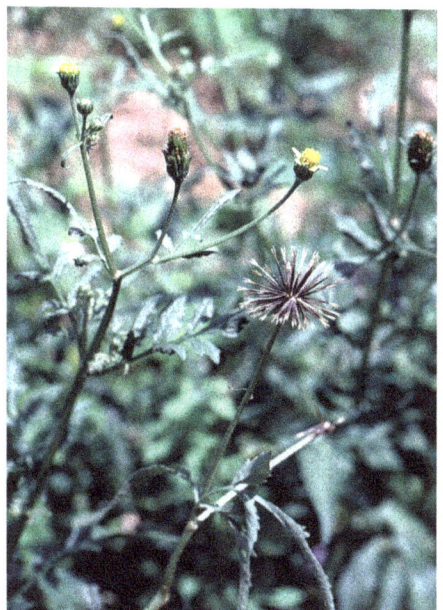

Duppy Needles, Monkey Needles, Spanish Needles

Bidens pilosa L.
Duppy Needles, Monkey Needles, Spanish Needles
Family: Asteraceae
Local Preparation: Hot infusion of the leaves.
Bioactive Chemical Profile: Flavonoids, polyacetylenic compounds (cytopiloyne) and tannins. (23, 47)
Pharmacological Activity: The methanolic extract of *B. pilosa* leaves prevented the establishment of hypertension and lowered elevated blood pressure in a hypertensive rat model. The decrease in systolic blood pressure was comparable to that of the nifedipine-treated control group. Blood pressure decreased by 17% and 21% at the dose of 75 and 150 mg/kg respectively. (47)

Ambrosia hispida Pursh.
Wild Geranium, Seaside Geranium
Family: Asteraceae
Local Preparation: Hot infusion or decoction of the leaves.
Bioactive Chemical Profile: Leaf extract has 84 essential oils with major constituents, borneol (19.4%) and spathulenol (11.8%). (48)
Pharmacological Activity: Borneol at a daily oral dose of 50 mg/kg biweekly can produce significant antihypertensive and antioxidant effect against L-NAME induced hypertensive rats. (49)

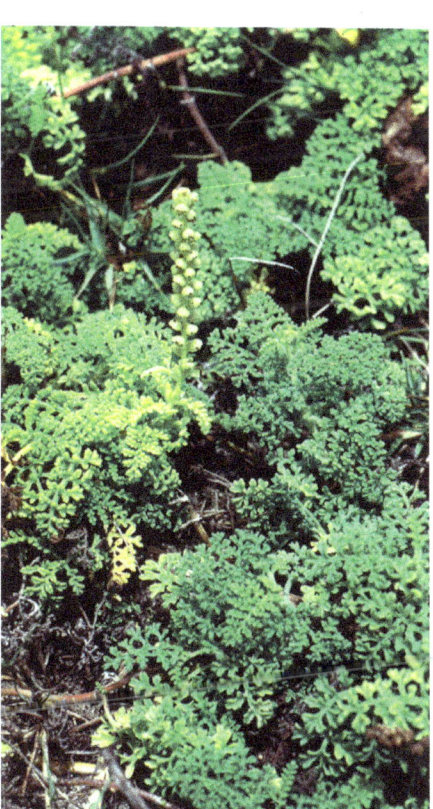

Wild Geranium, Seaside Geranium

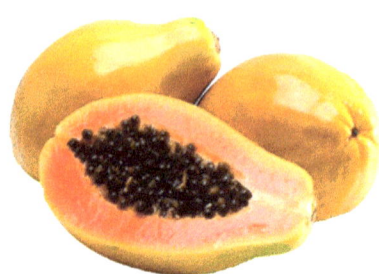
Pawpaw, Papaya

Carica papaya L. [DC011]
Pawpaw, Papaya
Family: Caricaceae
Local Preparation: Hot infusion of the leaves or fruit eaten. (2)
Bioactive Chemical Profile: Quercetin, ferulic acid and gallic acid. (50)
Pharmacological Activity: Papaya leaves in Nori preparation of 10% mixed with standard feed normalised both systolic and diastolic blood pressure and had a reduction in arterial stiffness in an animal model compared to the group receiving captopril, an established antihypertensive agent. (50, 51)

Cecropia schreberiana Miq.
Trumpet Tree, Pop-a-Gun
Family: Cecropiaceae
Local Preparation: Decoction of the leaves.
Bioactive Chemical Profile: Triterpenoids, flavonoids (flavone C-glycosides, flavanolignans and proanthocyanidins. (28)
Pharmacological Activity: Hypotensive effects were observed in

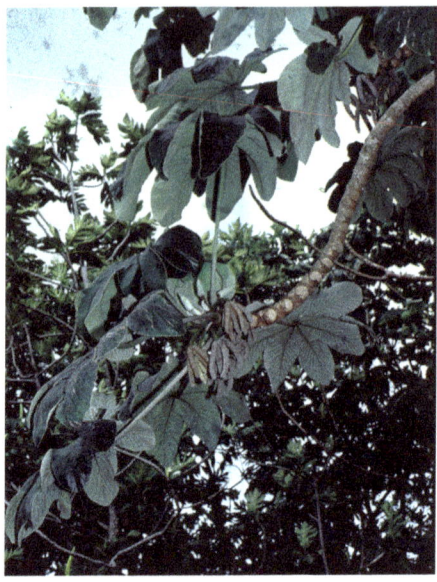
Trumpet Tree, Pop-a-Gun

animals treated with aqueous extracts of related species via blockade of type 1 calcium-channels on smooth muscles and an effect on β-2 adrenergic receptors. Dichloromethane/methanol and methanol extracts of the leaves inhibited Angiotensin Converting Enzyme (ACE) *in vitro*. (29)

Terminalia catappa L.
Barbados Almond, Seaside Almond
Family: Combretaceae
Local Preparation: Decoction of the leaves.
Bioactive Chemical Profile: Phenolic compounds (e.g. punicalagin), flavonoids and carotenoids. (52)
Pharmacological Activity: The phenolic-rich extracts showed remarkable enzyme inhibition activity *in vitro* with IC_{50} values in

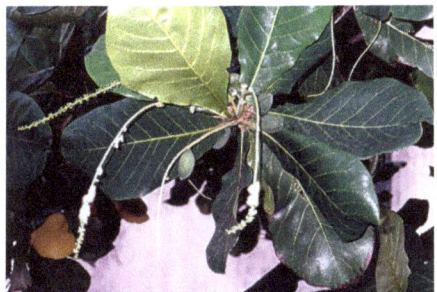
Barbados Almond, Seaside Almond

leaves and bark against Arginase [51.65 ± 2.57 (leaves); 53.91 ± 4.03 (bark)], Phosphodiesterase [238.44 ± 3.57 (leaves); 273.43 ± 4.03(bark)], Angiotensin Converting Enzyme (ACE) [64.74 ± 1.57 (leaves); 57.29 ± 2.03(bark)] with high antioxidant activities. (52, 53)

Momordica charantia L.[DC002]
Cerasee, Miraculous Vine, Crapaud, Pumpkin, Lizard Food
Family: Cucurbitaceae
Local Preparation: Hot infusion of the whole plant.
Bioactive Chemical Profile:
Proteins and peptides (momordins, momorcharins), terpenoids, saponins, flavonoids, phenolic compounds, essential oils and fatty acids. (30)
Pharmacological Activity: The extract of the whole plant normalized hypertension in a *dose dependent manner* in hypertensive Dahl salt-sensitive rats by acetylcholine mediated pathways. Also, the extracts of the whole plant reduced the Angiotensin Converting Enzyme (ACE) activities. Interestingly, a

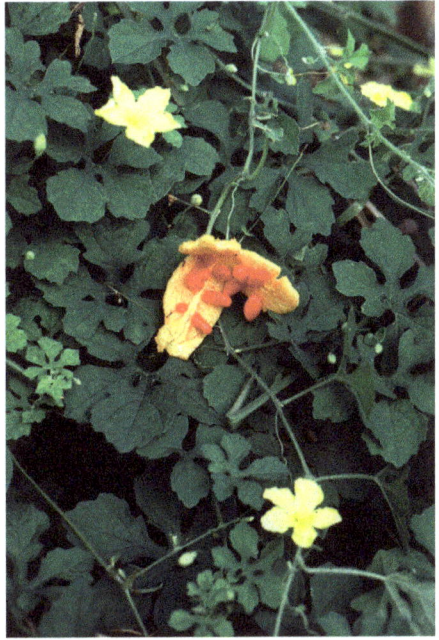
Cerasee, Miraculous Vine, Crapaud, Pumpkin, Lizard Food

preliminary open-label uncontrolled supplementation trial among 42 participants supplemented with 4.8 g lyophilized encapsulated *M. charantia* powder, administered daily for three months, showed no significant effects on high blood pressure, heart rate, and other parameters of the metabolic syndrome. (30, 31)

Phyllanthus amarus Schum.
Seed-Under-Leaf
Family: Euphorbiacae
Local Preparation: Hot infusion of the stem and leaves.
Bioactive Chemical Profile:
Lignans, flavonoids, hydrolysable tannins (ellagitannins), polyphenols, triterpenes, sterols and alkaloids. (9)

MEDICINAL PLANTS OF BARBADOS

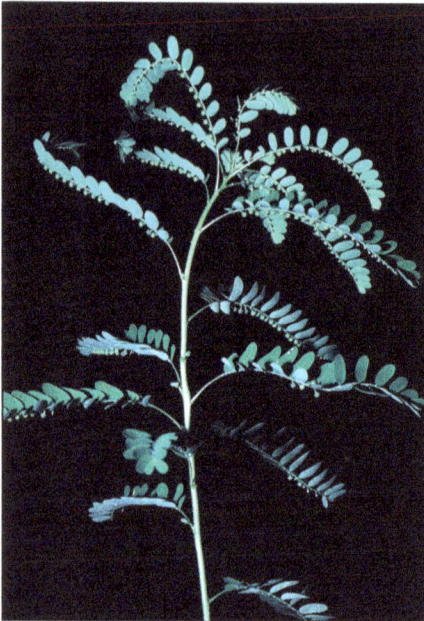

Seed-Under-Leaf

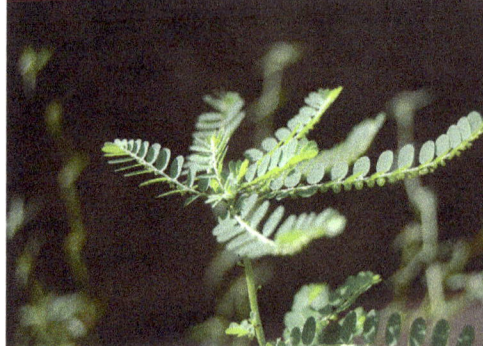

Seed-Under-Leaf

Pharmacological Activity: Anti-inflammatory, antioxidant and hypolipidemic effects have been reported. (9, 54) Treatments with the aqueous extract of the whole plant, *P. amarus* was administered by oral gavage at 100 and 300 mg/kg daily and prevented increase in systolic blood pressure, improved cardiac structure/function, and improved endothelial function in a deoxycorticosterone acetate (DOCA) salt induced hypertension model. (55)

Phyllanthus niruri L.
Seed-Under-Leaf
Family: Euphorbiacae
Local Preparation: Hot infusion of the stem and leaves.

Bioactive Chemical Profile: Flavonoids, alkaloids, terpenoids, lignans, polyphenols, tannins, coumarins and saponins. (32)
Pharmacological Activity: Anti-inflammatory, antioxidant and hypolipidemic effects have been reported. (32) *P. niruri* extracts showed a significant decrease in blood pressure (BP) of spontaneous hypertensive rats when compared to the baseline with the petroleum ether extract being the most potent. The extracts administered at a dose of 0.125–4 mg/ml daily by oral gavage also induced vasorelaxation on the endothelium-intact aorta ring of the treated rats. (56)

Desmodium incanum DC.
Sweetheart Bush
Family: Fabaceae
Local Preparation: Hot infusion of the plant.
Bioactive Chemical Profile: Flavonoids, alkaloids, terpenoids,

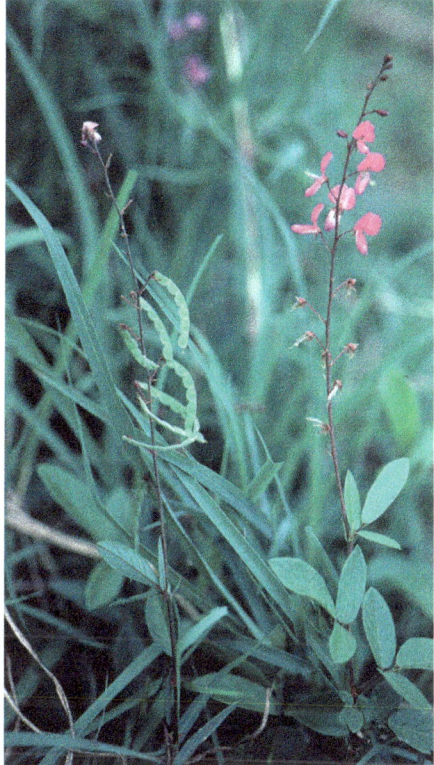
Sweetheart Bush

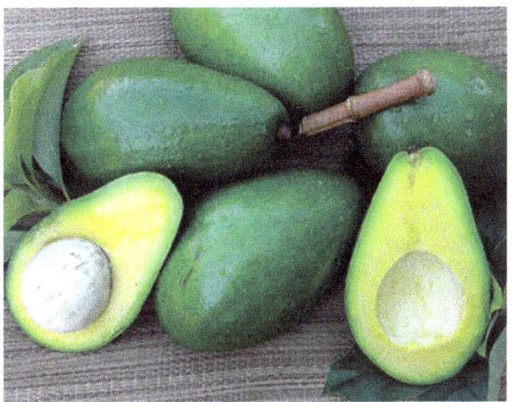
Pear

steroids, phenols, phenylpropanoids, glycosides and a number of volatile oils. (57)
Pharmacological Activity: Related species with similar phytochemical profiles have been reported to have anti-inflammatory, anti-oxidant and cardio-protective effects. (57)

Persea americana Mill.
Pear
Family: Lauraceae
Local Preparation: Hot infusion of the leaves, bottled and cooled overnight before drinking. (2)

Bioactive Chemical Profile: Alkanols, terpenoid glycosides, various furan ring-containing derivatives, flavonoids and a coumarin. (249)
Pharmacological Activity: Dose-related hypotensive effects were noted at the dose range of 6.25–50 mg/kg of the leaf aqueous and methanol extracts via intra-peritoneal injection on normotensive anesthetized rats. Doses above 12.5 mg/kg showed hypotensive effects which were significantly different from those on the control. (249)

Thespesia populnea (L.) Sol. ex Correa
Mahoe, Anodyne
Family: Malvaceae
Local Preparation: Hot infusion of the leaves.
Bioactive Chemical Profile: Carbohydrate, protein, tannins, phenol, glycosides, flavonoids, terpenes, saponins and mucilage in

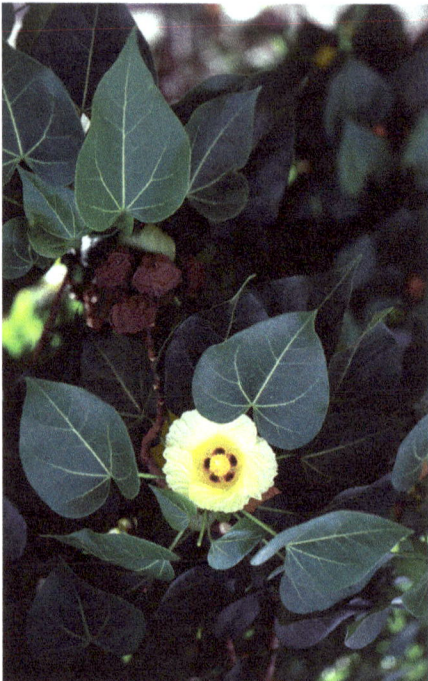

Mahoe, Anodyne

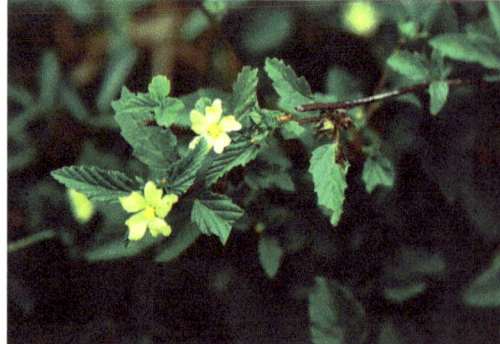

Broomweed

aqueous and ethanolic extracts of the bark. (58)
Pharmacological Activity: Administration of aqueous and methanolic extracts of *T. populnea* at a dose of 500 mg/kg resulted in significant free radical scavenging activity (potent antioxidant properties) in carbon tetrachloride-induced liver injury in rats. Various solvent extracts promoted diuretic activities at a dose of 400 mg/kg in albino rats. (58, 59).

Sida acuta Burm.f.
Broomweed
Family: Malvaceae
Local Preparation: Hot infusion of the leaves.

Bioactive Chemical Profile: Cryptolepine and quindolinone. (60)
Pharmacological Activity: Cryptolepine and quindolinine (10^{-12}–10^3 M), isolated from a related species (*S. rhombifolia*) resulted in significant vasorelaxation in mesenteric arteries of rats contracted with phenylephrine *in vitro*. (60)

Azadirachta indica A.Juss.
Neem
Family: Meliaceae
Local Preparation: Decoction of the leaves. (2)
Bioactive Chemical Profile: Nimbin, nimbidin, quercetin, limonoids, terpenoids, sterols, fatty acids, coumarins, azadiradione, hydrocarbons, sulphur containing compounds and phenolics. (34, 35)
Pharmacological Activity: An *A. indica* infused yogurt extract demonstrated antioxidant activity and maximum inhibition on Angiotensin Converting Enzyme (ACE) at 79.70 ± 11.2% *in vitro*. (37)

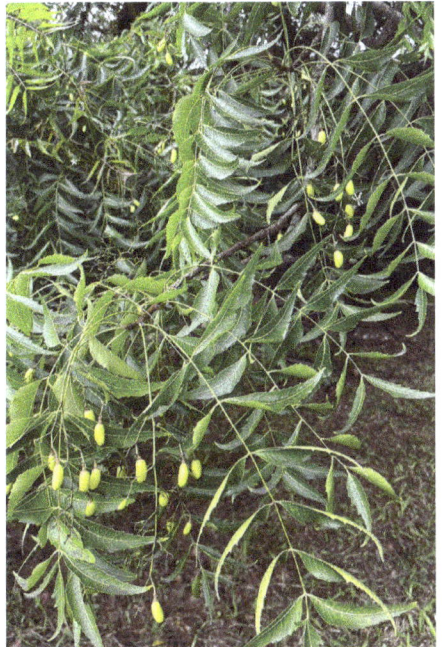
Neem

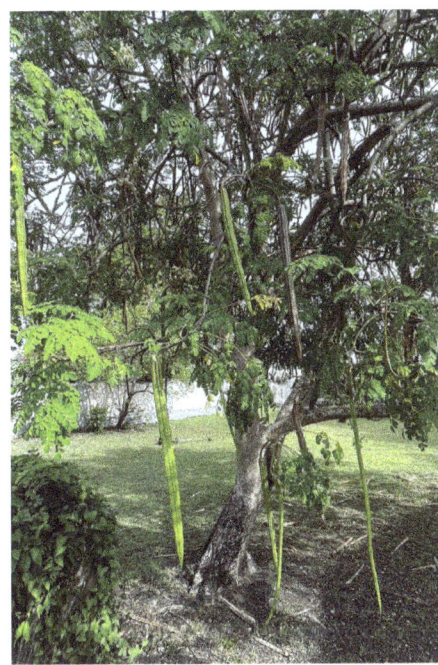
Moringa

Moringa oleifera Lam.
Moringa
Family: Moringaceae
Local Preparation: Decoction of the leaves. (2)
Bioactive Chemical Profile: Isoquercetin, catechin and tannic acid. (61)
Pharmacological Activity: The aqueous extract of the leaves administered daily at 30 and 60 mg/kg orally produced an antihypertensive effect in N(G)-nitro-L-arginine-methyl ester (L-NAME) hypertensive rats which may be mediated by alleviating vascular dysfunction, oxidative stress and promoting endothelium-dependent vasorelaxation. (61)

Bontia daphnoides L.
Wild Olive
Family: Myoporaceae
Local Preparation: Hot infusion of the leaves.
Bioactive Chemical Profile: Phytochemical analysis of the volatile constituents of *B. daphnoides'* leaves revealed the presence of 38 compounds. The major consitituents were dehydroepingaione (83.6%), an oxygenated sesquiterpene, represented the major constituent followed by alloaromadendrene (10.37%) and 2,3'-bifuran, 2,3,4,5-tetrahydro-5-methyl-5-[(4-methyl-2-furanyl)methyl] (2.14%). These may be limited in the infused aqueous extract but may still have some relevance. (250)

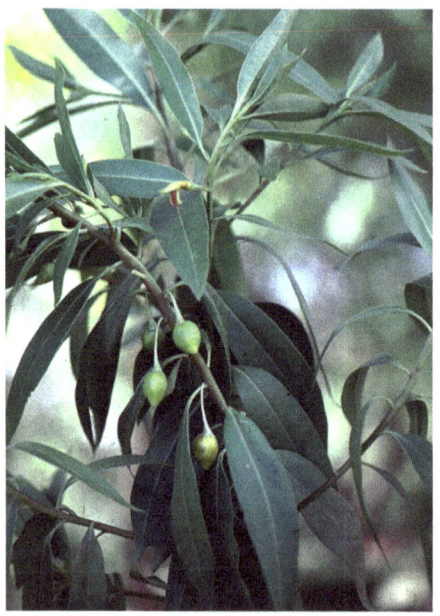
Wild Olive

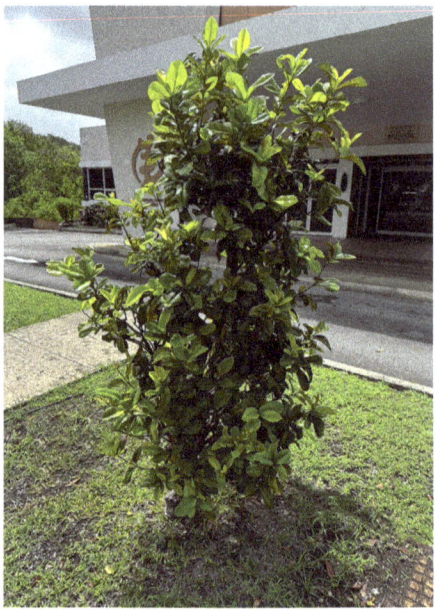
Bay Leaf

Pharmacological Activity: No preclinical / clinical studies were identified which validated hypotensive effects at the time of the literature assessment.

Pimenta racemosa (Mill.) J.W. Moore [DC018]
Bay Leaf
Family: Myrtaceae
Local Preparation: Hot infusion of the leaves, bottled and cooled overnight before drinking. (2)
Bioactive Chemical Profile: Terpenoids, steroids, saponins, phenolic nuclei, glycosides, tannins and quinines. (62)
Pharmacological Activity: The aqueous methanol extract (AME) of leaves showed significant free radical scavenging activity, SC_{50} = 4.6 µg/ml, using the 2, 2-diphenyl-1-picrylhydrazyl (DPPH) radical scavenging method. Anti-inflammatory effects of the extract were also confirmed which could contribute to cardio-protective effects. (62, 63)

Passiflora laurifolia L.
Water Lemon (1)
Family: Passifloraceae
Local Preparation: Hot infusion of the leaves.
Bioactive Chemical Profile: Passiflora species contain harmala alkaloids, harmane (passaflorine), harmine (telepathine), harmaline, harmol, harmalol and polyphenol (luteolin). (64)
Pharmacological Activity: Orally administered methanol extract

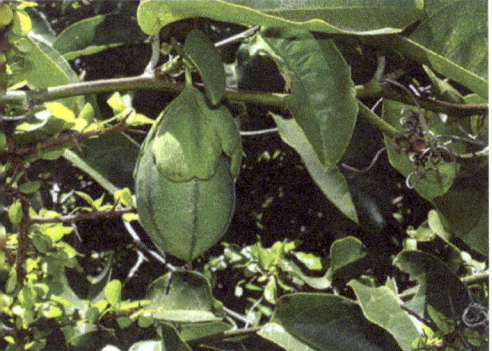

Water Lemon

of the rind of *Passiflora edulis,* an allied species of Passiflora at 10 mg/kg or 50 mg/kg or luteolin 50 mg/kg significantly lowered systolic blood pressure in spontaneously hypertensive rats. (64, 65)

Peperomia pellucida (L.) Kunth
Shine Bush
Family: Piperaceae
Local Preparation: Hot infusion of the leaves.
Bioactive Chemical Profile: Alkaloids (secolignans), tetrahydrofuran lignans, methoxylated dihydronaphthalenon, peperomins A, B, C, and E, sesamin and isoswertisin. (66)
Pharmacological Activity: Intravenous administration of *P. pellucida* aqueous extract at 10–30 mg/kg in normotensive rats led to dose-dependent hypotensive, bradycardic and vasorelaxant effects which may be mediated through nitric oxide-dependent mechanisms. Inhibitory effects of the extract on Angiotensin Converting Enzyme (ACE) are also noted. (66, 67)

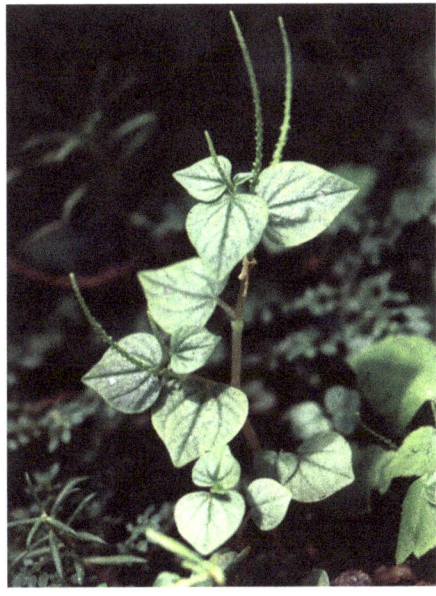

Shine Bush

Plantago major L.
English Plantain
Family: Plantaginaceae
Local Preparation: Hot infusion of the leaves.

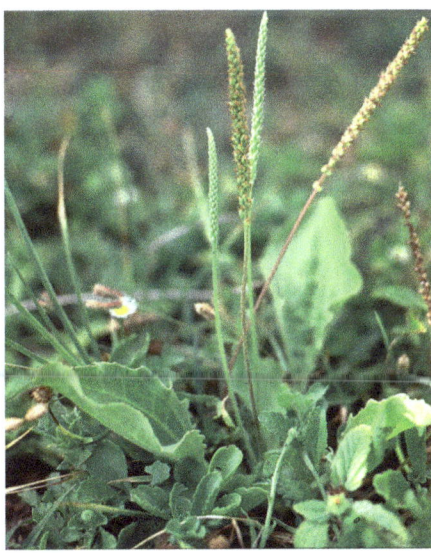

English Plantain

Bioactive Chemical Profile: Flavonoids, polysaccharides, terpenoids, lipids, iridoid glycosides, coumarins, mucilage and caffeic acid derivatives. (68)
Pharmacological Activity: Antilipidemic, anti-inflammatory and antioxidant effects have been reported along with an antihypertensive effect of the whole plant on mild to moderate hypertensive patients. (68, 69)

Spermacoce assurgens Ruiz & Pavon
Buttonweed
Family: Rubiaceae
Local Preparation: Hot infusion of the plant.
Bioactive Chemical Profile: Alkaloids, iridoids, flavonoids, and terpenoids are the main groups of constituents. Among them, alkaloids and iridoids are the main bioactive compounds in *in vivo* or *in vitro* studies. (251)
Pharmacological Activity: Anti-anflammatory, anti-oxidant and antihyperlipidemic effects have been noted among the Spermacoce genus. (251)

Scoparia dulcis L. (81)
Sweet Broom, Licorice Weed
Family: Scrophulariaceae
Local Preparation: Hot infusion of the plant.
Bioactive Chemical Profile: Scoparic acid, scopadulcic acid, scopadulciol, scopadulin, scoparinol and ammelinare and catecholamines. (70)
Pharmacological Activity: Ethanolic leaf and aqueous plant extracts of the plant reported to have anti-inflammatory, antioxidant and anti-hyperlipidemic effects respectively. Scoparinol has demonstrated diuretic activity *in vivo*. However, an aqueous fraction of *S. dulcis* revealed the presence of 2 catecholamines, noradrenaline and adrenaline, that may account for hypertensive and inotropic effects after parenteral administration. (70, 71).

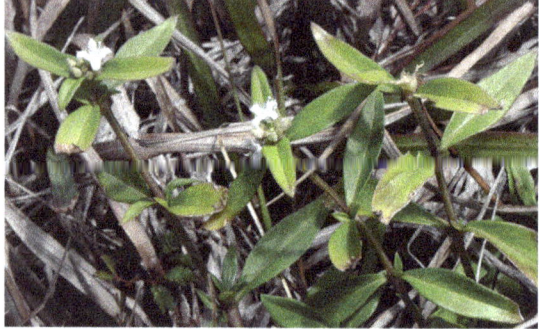
Buttonweed

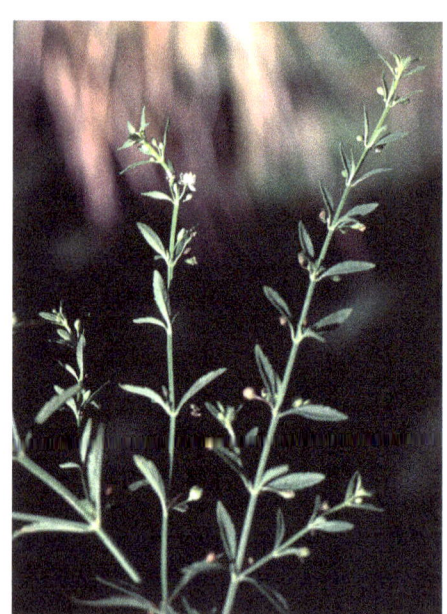
Sweet Broom, Licorice Weed

Physalis angulata L.
Cow Pops, Poppers
Family: Solanaceae
Local Preparation: Hot infusion or decoction of the leaves or an extraction of the berries.
Bioactive Chemical Profile:
Physalins, withanolides, flavonol glycoside and oleonolic acid. (72)
Pharmacological Activity: The methanolic leaf extract of *Physalis angulata L* administered orally at doses of 250, 500 and 1000 mg/kg produced a notable diuretic effect which appeared to be comparable to furosemide, an established diuretic agent, in rats. (73)

Laportea aestuans (L.) Chew
Nettle (1)
Family: Urticaceae
Local Preparation: Hot infusion of the leaves.
Bioactive Chemical Profile:
Saponins, tannins, flavanoids, phlobatanins and cardiac glycosides. (74)
Pharmacological Activity: The ethanolic extract of *L. aestuans* has weak antioxidant activity, i.e., IC_{50} of 554.30 µg/ml using the 2, 2-diphenyl-1-picrylhydrazyl (DPPH) radical scavenging method. At an oral dose of 0.6g/kg, 39.62% anti-inflammatory activity was reported using a rat carrageen-induced paw edema inflammatory model. (74)

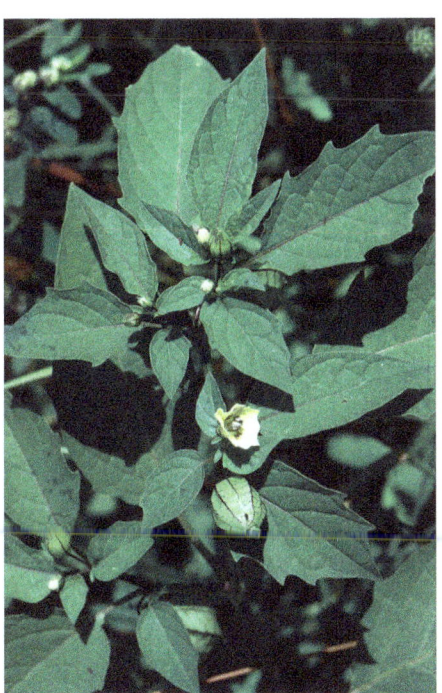

Cow Pops, Poppers

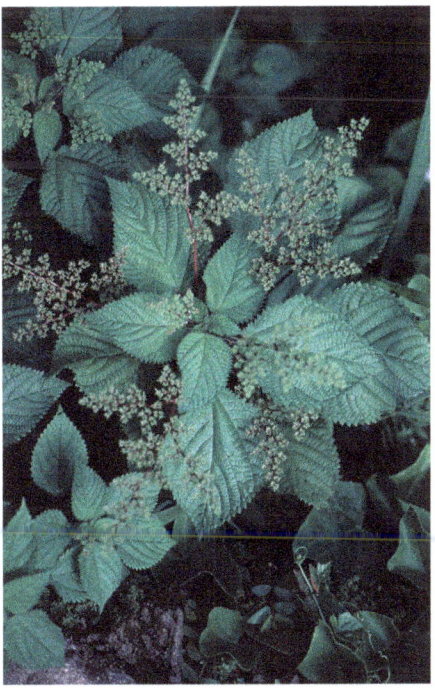

Nettle

MEDICINAL PLANTS OF BARBADOS

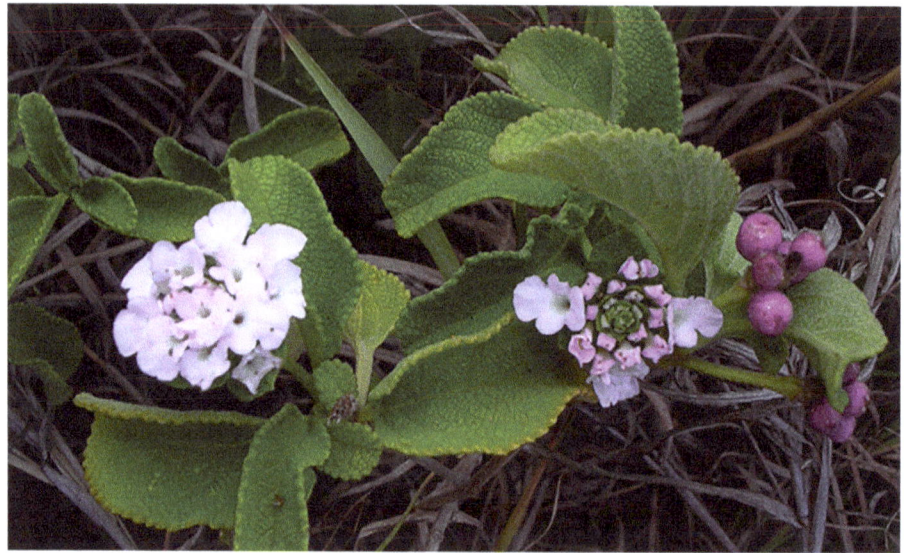

Rock Sage, Wild Sage

Lantana involucrata L.
Rock Sage, Wild Sage
Family: Verbenaceae
Local Preparation: Hot infusion of tea of the leaves.
Bioactive Chemical Profile: Alkaloids and sesquiterpenoids. (75, 76)
Pharmacological Activity: Alkaloid fraction of *L. camara* (related species) was shown to lower blood pressure in dogs. (75)

Aegiphila martinicensis Jacq.
Spirit Weed
Family: Verbenaceae
Local Preparation: Hot infusion of the shoots.
Bioactive Chemical Profile: No bioactive compounds and pharmacological study have been identified in alignment with traditional use.

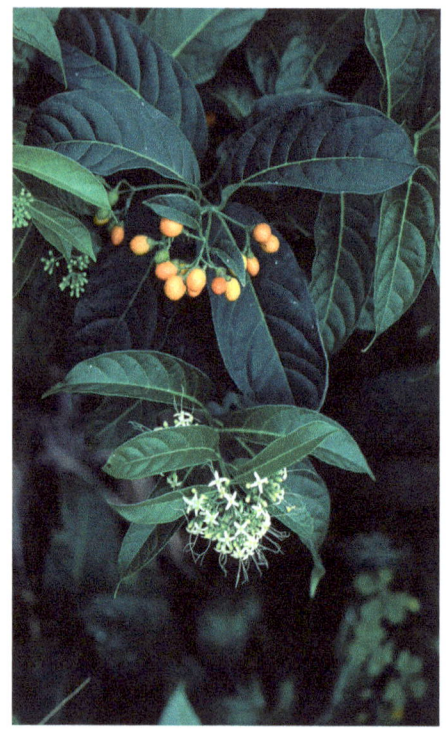

Spirit weed

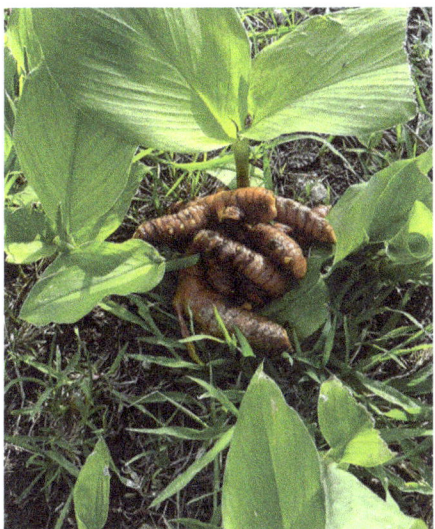

Turmeric

Curcuma longa L.
Turmeric
Family: Zingiberaceae
Local Preparation: Boiled rhizomes, or mixed with black pepper in hot water. (2)
Bioactive Chemical Profile: Curcumin, demethoxycurcumin and tetrahydrocurcumin. (77)
Pharmacological Activity: Studies in male normotensive rats have reported the effectiveness of the methanolic extract of *C. longa* as a hypotensive and vasorelaxant agent with a significant reduction in mean arterial pressure at a dose range of 20 mg/kg and 30 mg/kg orally. These effects have been associated with *C. longa's* antioxidant, anti-inflammatory activity, calcium (II) ion concentration interference, β2-adrenergic receptor activation, and renin-angiotensin-aldosterone system inhibition activities. (77)

NEURODEGENERATIVE DISEASES

Synedrella nodiflora (L.) Gaertn.
Porter bush
Family: Asteraceae
Local Preparation: Hot infusion of the leaves.
Bioactive Chemical Profile: Flavonoids, steroids, triterpenoids, saponins, alkaloids and phytosterols. (78)
Pharmacological Activity: Petroleum ether leaf extract produced cerebroprotective effects in global cerebral ischemia in rats by reducing hyperlocomotion and neuronal damage. (78)

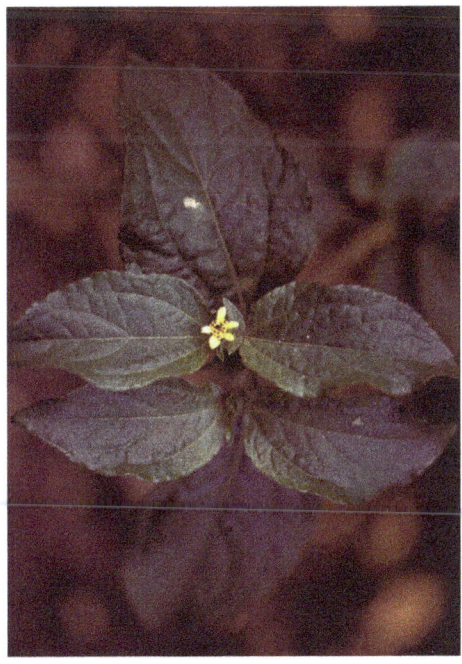

Porter bush

BARBADIAN MEDICINAL PLANTS USED IN THE TREATMENT OF COMMUNICABLE DISEASES

BACTERIAL INFECTIONS – SKIN/TOPICAL AILMENTS

Amaranthus dubius C. Matius
Spinach (1)
Family: Amaranthacae
Local Preparation: Poultice of the leaves with olive oil for skin ailments. A decoction of the plant to clean wounds.
Bioactive Chemical Profile:
Flavonoids, steroids, terpenoids and cardiac glycosides were commonly found in leaf extracts of three related species. (79)

Pharmacological Activity: The leaf extracts of three related plant species *Amaranthus hybridus, Amaranthus spinosus* and *Amaranthus caudatus* demonstrated dose dependent antimicrobial activity against the gram- positive *Staphylococcus aureus* and *Bacillus spp,* gram- negative *Escherichia coli, Salmonella typhi, Pseudomonas aeruginosae, Proteus mirabillis* and *Klebsiella pneumoniae*. The minimum inhibitory concentration exhibited by *A. spinosus* extracts against the *S. typhi* was 129 mg/ml. The MIC of the *A. hybridus* extracts against the tested organisms ranged between 200 and 755 mg/ml whereas that of *A. caudatus* was between 162.2 and 665 mg/ml. (70, 80)

Allium sativum L.
Garlic
Family: Amaryllidaceae
Local Preparation: Ingested raw for cuts and sores. (2)

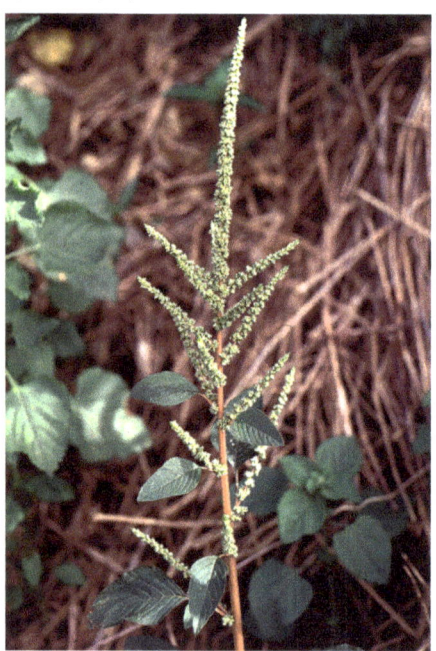
Spinach

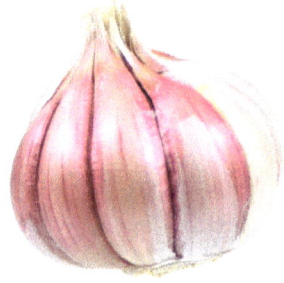
Garlic

Bioactive Chemical Profile: Allicin, diallyl sulfide and alliin. (81)
Pharmacological Activity: Antioxidant, anti-inflammatory, and anti-microbial properties have been verified by numerous studies. Raw garlic has anti-bacterial effects against *H. pylori* residing in the stomach and can be taken with routine drugs for the treatment of gastric *H. pylori* infection. (82, 83)

Hymenocallis caribaea (L. emend. Gawl.) Herbert
Spider Lily, Wild Garlic
Family: Amaryllidaceae
Local Preparation: Crushed bulbs used for lesions and burns.
Bioactive Chemical Profile: Alkaloids, flavonoids, glycosides, terpenes, terpenoids and phenolics have been identified in the methanolic extract of the leaves of a related species, *Hymenocallis littoralis*. (84, 85)
Pharmacological Activity: Antibiofilm and antimicrobial activities were confirmed against *S. aureus* NCIM 2654 with a minimum inhibitory concentration of 45 mg/ml for the methanolic extract of *H. littoralis*. Alkaloids extracted from the bulb of a related species, *H. littoralis*, possess anti-viral, anti-neoplastic and cytotoxic properties. (84)

Hippeastrum puniceum (Lam.) Ktze.
Easter Lily, Barbados Lily, Amaryllis
Family: Amaryllidaceae
Local Preparation: Crushed bulbs used for ailments.
Bioactive Chemical Profile: Alkaloids (3-O-Acetyl-narcissidine). (86)
Pharmacological Activity: Leaf extracts of the related species *H. fosteri* have exhibited dose dependent antimicrobial activity against Gram positive *Bacillus subtilis, Staphylococcus aureus* and *Escherichia coli;* and Gram negative *Klebsiella pneumoniae*. (87)

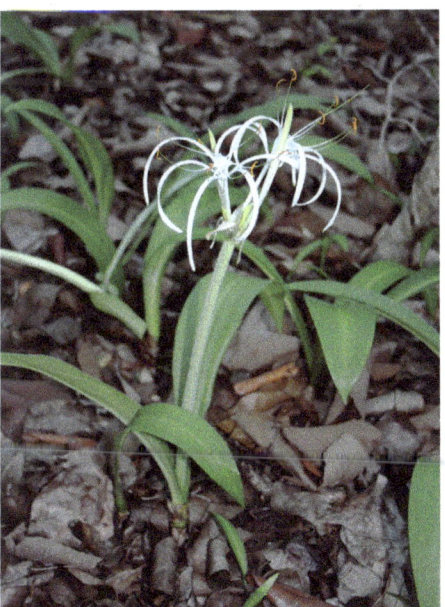

Spider Lily, Wild Garlic

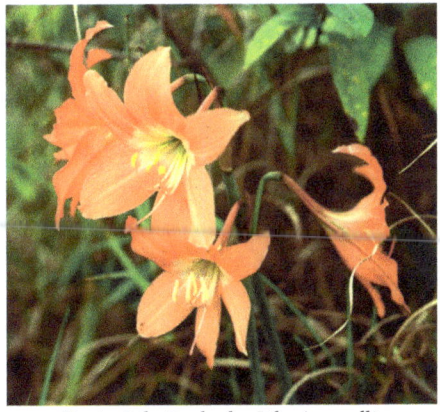

Easter Lily, Barbados Lily, Amaryllis

Aloe vera (L.) Burm.f. [DC009]
Aloes
Family: Asphodelaceae
Local Preparation: Cut open and rubbed on wounds and sores. (2)
Bioactive Chemical Profile: Anthraquinones (aloe emodin, aloetic acid, alovin, anthracine), saponins (glycosides) and steroids (lupenol). (88)
Pharmacological Activity: Studies have demonstrated that the anthraquinones, saponins and steroids have antibacterial and antiseptic activities. (88)

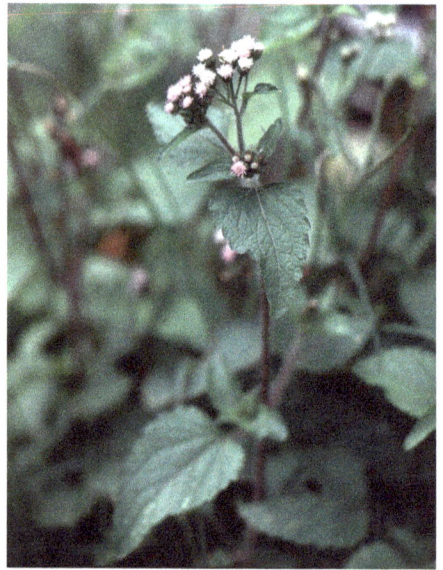

Wild Ageratum

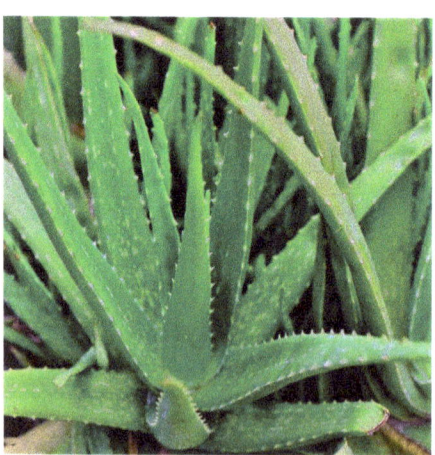

Aloes

Ageratum conyzoides L.
Wild Ageratum
Family: Asteraceae
Local Preparation: Poultice of the leaves for sores.
Bioactive Chemical Profile: Alkaloids, coumarins, flavonoids, chromenes, benzofurans, sterols and terpenoids. (89)
Pharmacological Activity: Antibacterial activity of the aqueous extract showed a significant control of the growth of *A. viscolactis, K. aerogenes, B. cereus* and *S. pyogenes*. The essential oil obtained from the plant showed antibacterial activity against *V. cholerae, S. shigae, S. pyogenes, C. diphtheriae* and *S. typhi*. (89, 90)

Bidens pilosa L.
Duppy Needles, Monkey Needles, Spanish Needles
Family: Asteraceae
Local Preparation: Hot infusion of the leaves.
Bioactive Chemical Profile: Flavonoids, polyacetylenic compounds (cytopiloyne), terpenoids, steroids and tannins. (23, 47, 91)
Pharmacological Activity: The dichloromethane extracts of *B. pilosa* demonstrated high antibacterial

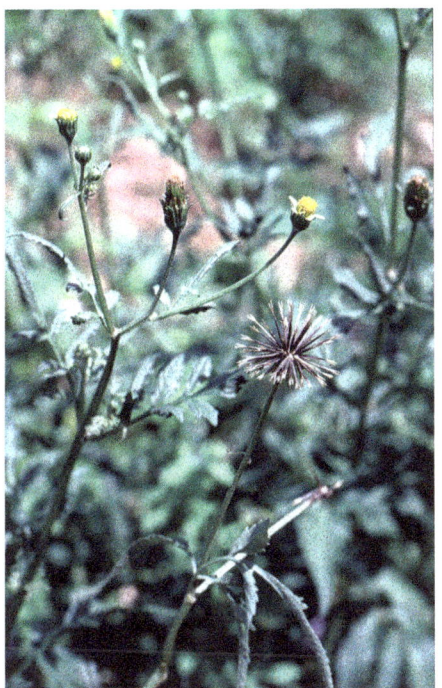

Duppy Needles, Monkey Needles, Spanish Needles

Sphagneticola trilobata (L.) Pruski [DC010]

Carpet Daisy, Lad Love, Wedelia
Family: Asteraceae
Local Preparation: Decoction of the shoot, and an extract of the leaves or a poultice of leaves for sores.
Bioactive Chemical Profile: Crude hydroalcoholic extract from leaves of *S. trilobata* revealed the presence of phenolic compounds, anthracene derivatives, and mono-, sesqui-, and diterpenes. Kaurenoic acid is also a phytoconstituent. (92, 93)
Pharmacological Activity: The crude hydroalcoholic extract from leaves of S. *trilobata* demonstrated antibacterial activity against multiple bacterial strains. For e.g., *Staphylococcus aureus* (ATCC25923) and *Staphylococcus spp.* (MRSA 9606) with a minimum inhibitory concentration of 3,125 µg/ml and 6,250 mg/ml respectively as well as antinociceptive effects during pain. (92, 94)

activity against *Klebsiella pneumoniae*, commercial probiotics (combination of *Lactobacillus acidophilus, Lactobacillus casei, Lactobacillus plantarum, Lactobacillus rhamnosus, Lactobacillus salivarius, Lactobacillus bifidum, Lactobacillus breve, Lactobacillus lactis, and Lactobacillus thermophillus*), *E. coli* ATCC25922™, *Salmonella typhimurium* ATCC13311™, *Shigella boydii* ATCC9207™ and *Vibrio parahaemolyticus* ATCC17802™ with an average minimum inhibitory concentration of 0.56 mg/ml. Other extracts (acetone and methanol) produced better antioxidant and antibacterial activities. (91)

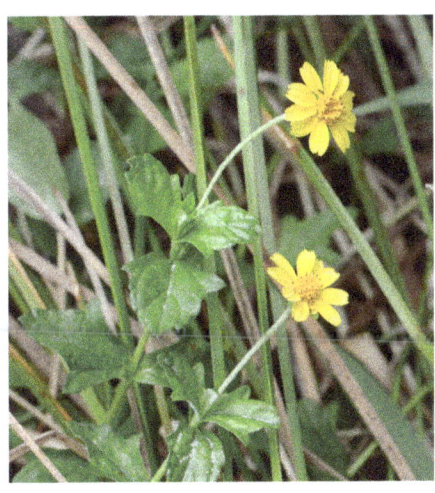

Carpet Daisy, Lad Love, Wedeliaa

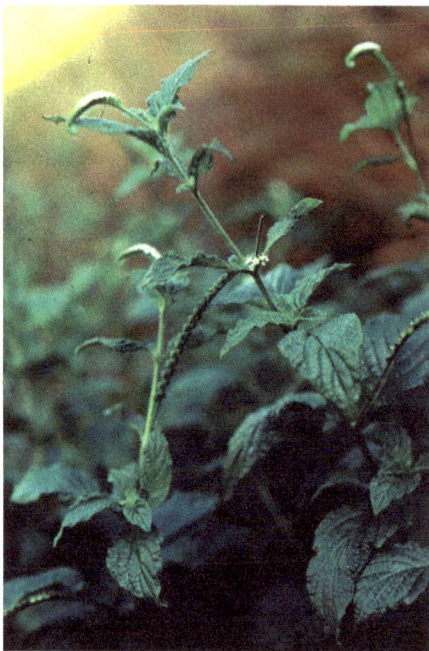
Wild Clary

Heliotropium angiospermum Murray
Wild Clary (1)
Family: Boraginaceae
Local Preparation: Decoction of the leaves.
Bioactive Chemical Profile: Pyrrolizidine alkaloids, phenolic compounds, terpenoids and quinones have been reported in species of genus Heliotropium. Examples of compounds with antibacterial activity among *Heliotropium* species are cycloartenone, b-amyrin, b-amyrin acetate, europine, lasiocarprine and b-sitosterol (95).
Pharmacological Activity: The methanolic extract of a related species, *H. bacciferum*, exhibited a significant antimicrobial activity against strains *Staphylococcus aureus, Bacillus cereus, Pseudomonas aeruginosa, Escherichia coli,* and *Salmonella enteritidis*. The chloroform and petroleum ether fractions of *H. bacciferum* inhibited the growth of *S. aureus, B. cereus* and *P. aeruginosa* with a minimum inhibitory concentration (MIC) of 15.625 μg/ml, *S. enteritidis* with 62.5 μg/ml and *E. coli* with 125 μg/ml respectively. Antimicrobial effects of other related species have also been reported. (95, 96)

Heliotropium indicum L
Wild Clary
Family: Boraginaceae
Local Preparation: Decoction of the leaves for applying to the skin or as a gargle for mouth ulcers.
Bioactive Chemical Profile: Heliotropium species comprise pyrrolizidine alkaloids, flavonoids and

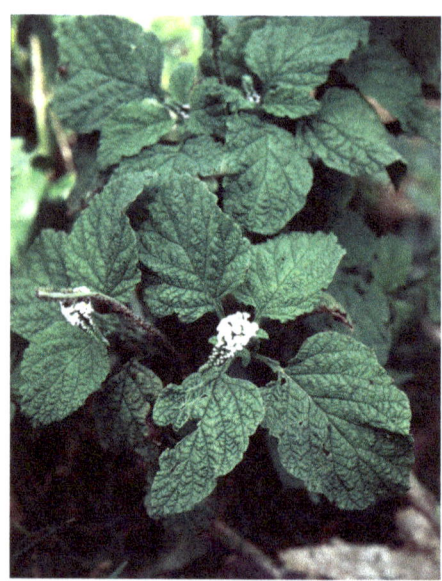
Wild Clary

terpenoids. (97) Also, note the above entry for *Heliotropium angiospermum* Murray.
Pharmacological Activity: Antimicrobial effects have been reported from extracts of the Heliotropium species. (97) Note the above entry for *Heliotropium angiospermum* Murray.

Tournefortia volubilis L.
Chigger Nut, Soldier Bush
Family: Boraginaceae
Local Preparation: Application of oil smeared leaves for sores.
Bioactive Chemical Profile: Terpenoids, salvianolic and caffeic acids are present in a closely related species, *T. sarmentosa*. (98, 99)
Pharmacological Activity: Caffeic and salvianolic acids (from *T. sarmentosa*) demonstrated ability to increase phagocytic uptake, inhibit bacterial survival within differentiated HL-60 leukemia cells and modulate neutrophil function. (98)

Carica papaya L. [DC011]
Pawpaw, Papaya
Family: Caricaceae
Local Preparation: Preparation of the seeds and fruit for boils. Poultice of the leaves can also be applied. (3)
Bioactive Chemical Profile: Oleic acid (antibacterial) and carpaine (wound-healing). (100, 101)
Pharmacological Activity: The antibacterial effect of oleic acid was determined in live fish, *Channa punctatus*, infected with pathogenic strains of *Klebsiella* PKBSG14 at a dose of 0.75 CFU/ml *in vivo*. Its effective antibacterial potential was reported at dose range of 0.5 mg/kg and 1 mg/kg administered biweekly and was assessed in relation to DNA fragmentation, comet tail length and toxicity biomarkers such as reactive oxygen species (ROS) generation in the pathogen. (101)

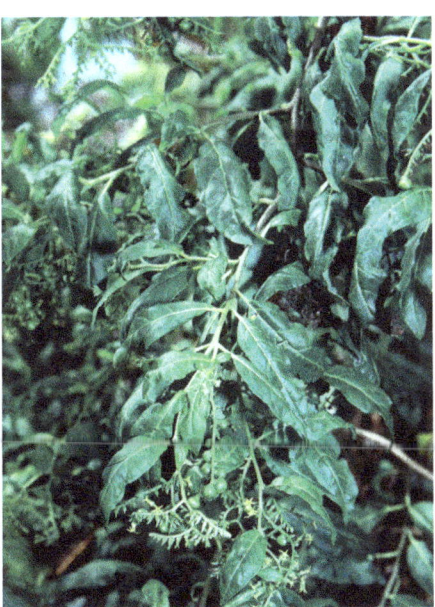

Chigger Nut, Soldier Bush

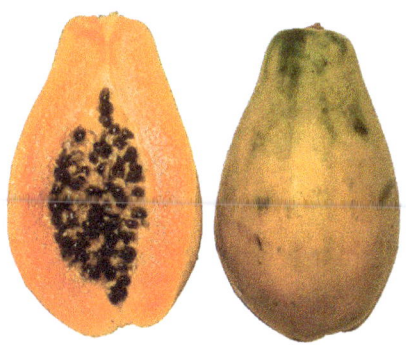

Pawpaw, Papaya

MEDICINAL PLANTS OF BARBADOS

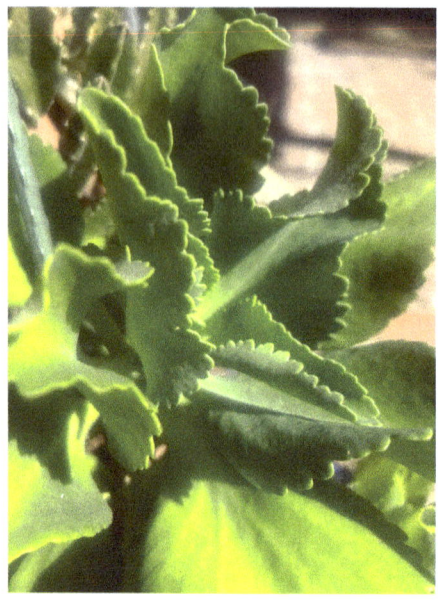

Wonder of the World

Cucumis sativus L.
Cucumber
Family: Cucurbitaceae
Local Preparation: Fruit slices placed on eyelids for sore eyes. (2)
Bioactive Chemical Profile: Alkaloids, anthocyanins, flavonoids, polyphenols, saponins and steroids. (106, 107)
Pharmacological Activity: The fruit's peel and pulp extracted with phosphate buffer saline (PBS) show antibacterial activity against *Staphylococcus aureus* and *Klebsiella pneumoniae* with an inhibition zone of 7.0±0 mm for both organisms. (106, 107)

Kalanchoe pinnata (Lam.) Pers. [DC005]
Wonder of the World
Family: Crassulaceae
Local Preparation: Leaves placed on wounds/sores. (2)
Bioactive Chemical Profile: Phenanthrene, squalene, phytol. (102, 103) Alkaloids, glycosides, carbohydrates, flavonoids, saponins, steroids, tannins, terpenoids and phenols. (104, 105)
Pharmacological Activity: Plant extracts inhibit inflammatory processes and bacterial growth. Methanolic extracts of the leaves were shown to specifically affect *Staphylococcus aureus, Pseudomonas aeruginosa* and *Escherichia coli*. The ethanolic extract of the leaves also accelerated wound healing. (104, 105)

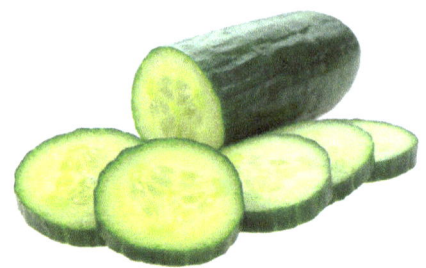

Cucumber

Vaccinium myrtillus L.
Bilberry
Family: Ericaceae
Local Preparation: A hot infusion of the leaves for sore eyes. (2)
Bioactive Chemical Profile: Hydroxycinnamic acids (esp. chlorogenic), hydrobenzoic acids, flavanols (gallic acid equivalents), hydroxycinnamic acids, proanthrocyandins and tannins. (108, 109)

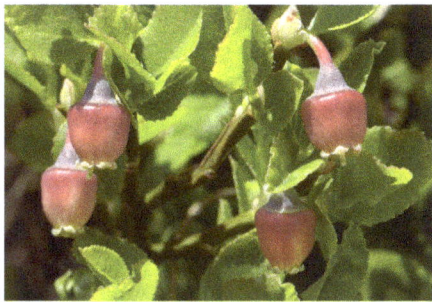
Bilberry

Pharmacological Activity: Significant antimicrobial effects of a polar extract (acetone and water) of the leaves against *Staphylococcus aureus* with a minimum inhibitory concentration 0.75–1.5 mg/ml has been documented. (109)

Jatropha curcas L.
Physic Nut, Monkey Fat Pork
Family: Euphorbiacae

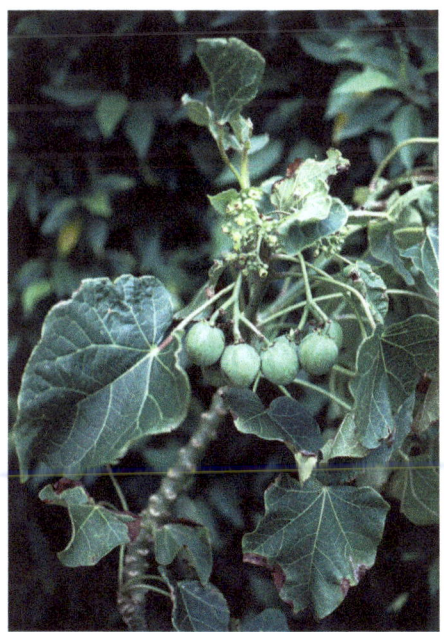
Physic Nut, Monkey Fat Pork

Local Preparation: Oil extracted from the seeds and applied to skin ailments. A leaf and sap preparation is also applied to bruises.

Bioactive Chemical Profile: Seeds' lipid composition includes triacylglycerols, diacylglycerols, monoacylglycerols, free fatty acids (linoleic acid, beheric acid & steric acid are major constituents), sterols and polar lipids. (110, 111)

Pharmacological Activity: The sap exhibited bactericidal actions against common bacteria species of *Staphylococcus, Bacillus* and *Micrococcus* species on contact and retained such effects on a treated laboratory bench surface for close to six hours after initial application. (110)

Chamaesyce hirta (L.) Millisp [DC016]
Milk Weed
Family: Euphorbiacae

Local Preparation: A preparation of the leaves or poultice for applying to sores.

Bioactive Chemical Profile: Triterpene and taraxerol have been isolated from the stems. Phytol and phytyl fatty acid esters have been yielded from the leaves and the roots contain cycloartenyl fatty acid ester, lupeol fatty acid ester, α-amyrin fatty acid ester and β-amyrin fatty acid ester, linoleic acid, β-sitosterol and squalene. (112) The ethanolic extract has been reported to contains tannins, flavonoids, alkaloids and cardiac glycosides. (113)

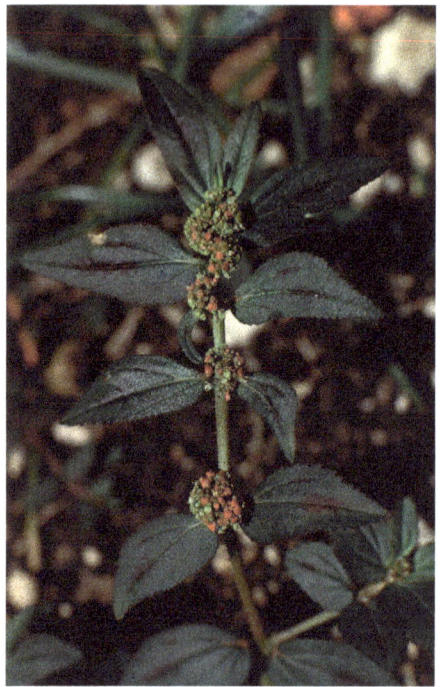
Milk weed

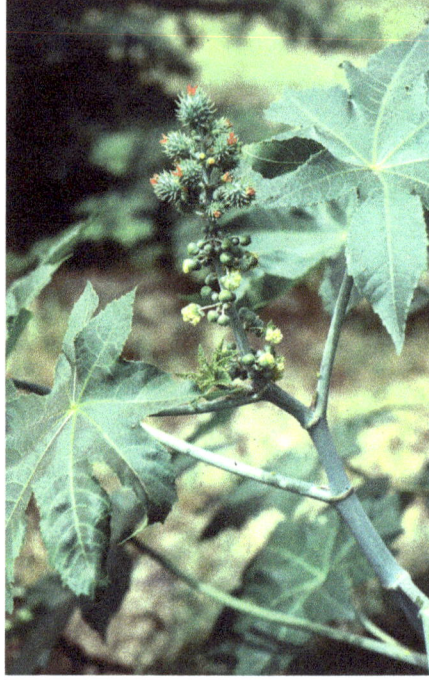
Castor Oil

Pharmacological Activity: Ethanolic extract of *E. hirta* (synonym) inhibited the growth of the *Escherichia coli, Staphylococcus aureus, Pseudomonas aeruginosa* and *Bacillus subtili* with minimum inhibitory concentrations of 58.09 mg/ml, 22.55 mg/ml, 57.64 mg/ml and 74.61 mg/ml respectively. (113)

Ricinus communis L. [DC004]
Castor Oil
Family: Euphorbiacae
Local Preparation: A preparation of the leaves or poultice for applying to sores.
Bioactive Chemical Profile: Overall phytochemical profile includes steroids, saponins, alkaloids, flavonoids and glycosides. The dried leaves of *R. communis* has two alkaloids (ricinine and N-demethylricinine), flavones and phenolic compounds. The leaf oil contains camphor and 1,8-cineole (known for antimicrobial activity). The seeds contain 45% of fixed oil (glycosides of ricinoleic, isoricinoleic, stearic and dihydroxystearic acids) lipases and a crystalline alkaloid, ricinine. (114)
Pharmacological Activity: The antimicrobial activities of *Ricinus communis* were good against dermatophytic and pathogenic bacterial strains *Streptococcus progenies* and *Staphylococcus aureus* as well as *Klebsiella pneumonia* and

Escherichia coli. Different solvent extracts of the roots of *Ricinus communis* possessed antimicrobial activity at a concentration of 200mg/ml using well diffusion method against pathogenic microorganisms such as *Escherichia coli, Staphylococcus aureus, Pseudomonas aeruginosa, Salmonella typhimurium, Proteus vulgaris* and *Bacillus subtili*s. The isolated leaf oil showed strong antimicrobial activity against all microorganisms tested with higher sensitivity for *Bacillus subtilis, Staphylococcus aureus* and *Enterobacter cloacae*. Minimum inhibitory concentrations ranged from 120 µg/ml to 300 µg/ml for the latter. (114, 115)

Azadirachta indica A.Juss.
Neem
Family: Meliaceae
Local Preparation: A decoction of the leaves for sore eyes. Pods applied to wounds. Poultice made from the leaf for applying to the affected area on the skin. (2, 3)

Bioactive Chemical Profile: Nimbin, nimbidin (antibacterial), quercetin, limonoids, terpenoids, sterols, fatty acids, coumarins, azadiradione, hydrocarbons, sulphur containing compounds and phenolics. (34, 35)
Pharmacological Activity: Neem oil has been shown to inhibit many strains of pathogenic bacteria such as *Staphylococcus aureus* in clinical trials. The oil from the leaves, seed and bark possesses a wide spectrum of antibacterial action against Gram-negative and Gram-positive microorganisms such as *Mycobacterium, Tuberculosis* and streptomycin resistant strains. Nimbidin has been reported to have antibacterial properties. (34, 35)

Pimenta racemosa (Mill.) J.W. Moore [DC018]
Bay Leaf
Family: Myrtaceae
Local Preparation: A decoction of leaves applied to soft tissue injuries. (3)
Bioactive Chemical Profile: Terpenoids, steroids, saponins, phenolic nuclei, glycosides, tannins,

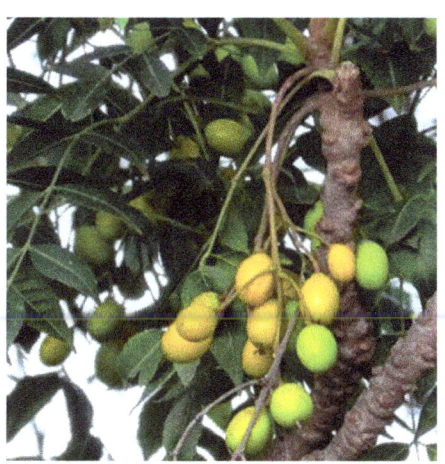

Neem

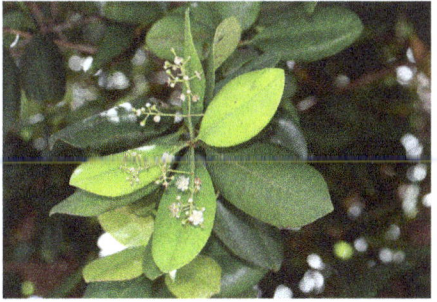

Bay Leaf

and quinines. 1,8-cineole, linalool and myrcene were noted as major constituents in the essential oils of the flower. (62, 116)

Pharmacological Activity: The antimicrobial effects of the essential oils of the flowers have been reported against *Bacillus subtilis, Geotrichum candidum, Staphylococcus aureus* and *Penicillium italicum* with minimum inhibitory concentrations ranging from 0.49–6.22 µg/ml. These effects were noted to be comparable to ampicillin and amphotericin B standards. (116)

Chiococca alba (L.) Hitchc
Snowberry, Tim-Tom Bush (1)
Family: Rubiaceae
Local Preparation: Decoction of the roots for sores and to treat urinogenital infections.

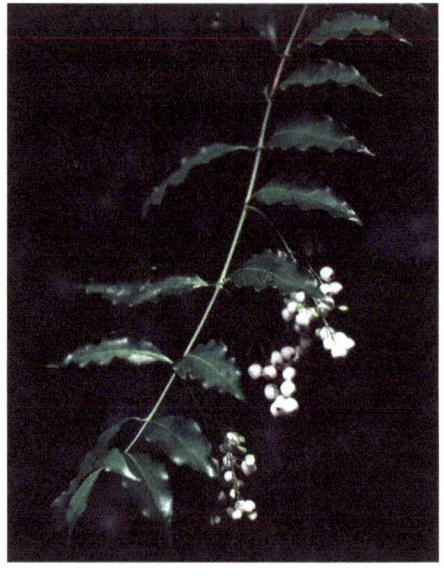

Snowberry, Tim-Tom Bush (detail)

Bioactive Chemical Profile: Two ent-kaurane diterpenes, 1-hydroxy-18-nor-kaur-4,16-dien-3-one and 15-hydroxy-kaur-16-en-3-one, along with the four known metabolites kaur-16-en-19-ol, kaurenoic acid, merilactone, and ribenone and a mixture of sterols (stigmasterol and β-sitosterol) were isolated from the ethanolic root extract of *Chiococca alba*. (117)

Pharmacological Activity: Anti-staphylococcal activity of ent-kaurene-type diterpenoids from the 5% methanolic extract of roots has been reported. (118)

Psychotria tenuifolia Sw.
Wild Coffee
Family: Rubiaceae
Local Preparation: A decoction of the leaves for applying to the skin.

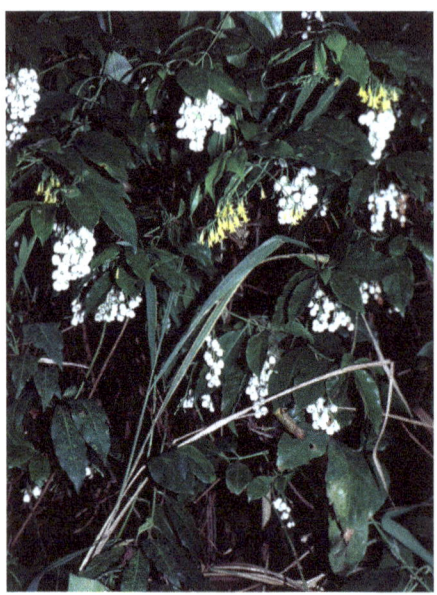

Snowberry, Tim-Tom Bush

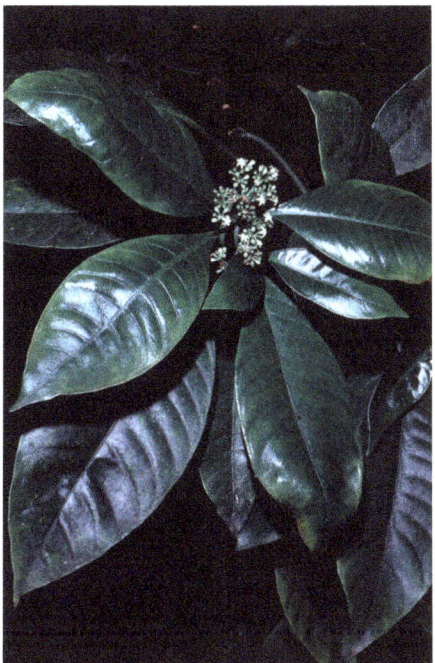

Wild Coffee

Bioactive Chemical Profile: The genus Psychotria's phytochemical profile includes alkaloids (indole, monoterpene indole, quinoline and isoquinoline), flavonoids, coumarins, terpenoids and cyclic peptides. (119)
Pharmacological Activity: Ten Psychotria species were reported to have antimicrobial effects against Mycobacterium. The compound quadrigemine B extracted from *P. rostrata* showed bactericidal activity against *Escherichia coli* and *Staphylococcus aureus*. Alkaloids (sychotrimine and psychopentamine) extracted from the leaves showed anti-bactericidal activity against resistant gram-positive bacteria *Bacillus subtilis* and *S. aureus*. (119)

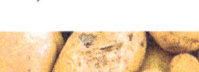*Solanum tuberosum* L.
English potato
Family: Solanaceae
Local Preparation: Potatoes soaked in water, water then mixed with castor oil and used to rinse eyes if sore. (2)
Bioactive Chemical Profile: Ferulic acid, caffeic acid and chlorogenic acid. (120)

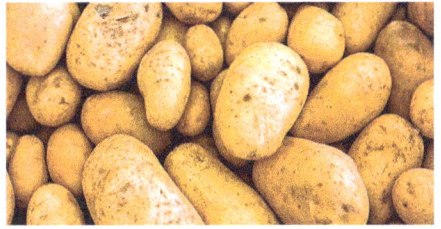

English potato

Pharmacological Activity: Potent antibacterial activity of the ethanolic extract of the peels were shown against both gram-positive *Staphylococcus aureus* and gram-negative *Pseudomonas aeruginosa* with minimum inhibitory concentrations of 0.62±0.00 mg/ml and 8.33±2.88 mg/ml respectively. (121)

Capraria biflora L.
West Indian Tea (1)
Family: Scrophulariaceae
Local Preparation: Decoction of the leaves as eyewash and for applying to wounds.
Bioactive Chemical Profile: Two chlorinated iridoids (3-hydroxymyopochlorin and 5-hydroxyglutinoside), five known iridoid glycosides, two flavonoid

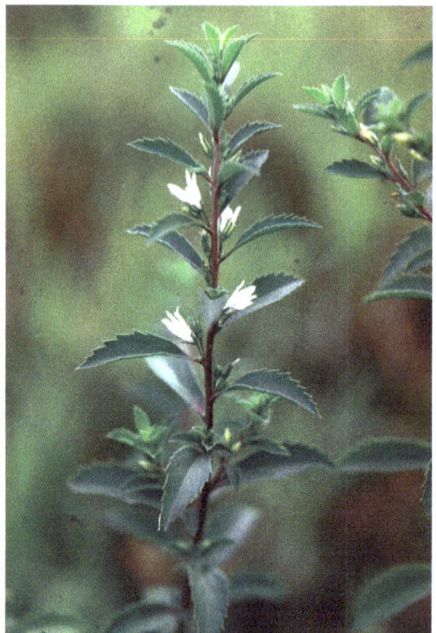
West Indian Tea

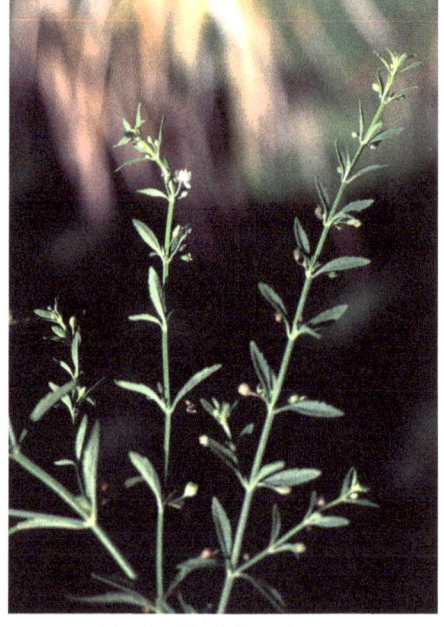
Licorice Weed, Sweet broom

glucuronides and the phenylethanoid glycoside, verbascoside were found in aerial parts of the plant. (122) An o-naphthoquinone, biflorin, has been isolated. (123)
Pharmacological Activity: Biflorin is an antibiotic compound with strong activity against Gram-positive and alcohol-acid resistant microbes. (123)

Scoparia dulcis L.
Licorice Weed, Sweet broom
Family: Scrophulariaceae
Local Preparation: Hot infusion of the leaves for sore throat and a preparation of the leaves or poultice for external sores.
Bioactive Chemical Profile: Coumarins, phenols, saponins, tannins, amino acids, flavonoids, terpenoids, diterpenoids, glycosides, steroids and catecholamines. (70, 124)
Pharmacological Activity: The methanolic extract of *S. dulcis* leaves showed antimicrobial effects against gram negative and positive bacteria. Zones of inhibition of 20 mm and 22 mm were exhibited against *E. coli* and *Staphylococcus aureus* respectively at a concentration of 500 µg/ml. (124, 125)

Curcuma longa L.
Turmeric
Family: Zingiberaceae
Local Preparation: Poultice of the leaves or roots and applied to cuts/wounds. (3)
Bioactive Chemical Profile: Curcuminioids. (126)
Pharmacological Activity: The

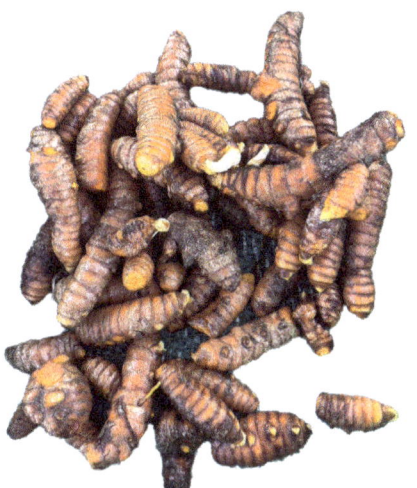
Turmeric

methanolic extract of the leaves of *Curcuma longa* shows antibacterial activity with a zone of inhibition of 14.65 mm between 10–12 hours of incubation against *Diplococcus pneumoneae, Streptococcus pyogens, Micrococcus glutamicus* and *Bacillus cereus* using the Disc Diffusion Susceptibility Method. (127, 128)

BACTERIAL INFECTIONS – RESPIRATORY AILMENTS

Aloe vera (L.) Burm.f. [DC009]
Aloes
Family: Asphodelaceae
Local Preparation: Eaten raw to help cough. (1)
Bioactive Chemical Profile: Acemannan, anthraquinones (aloe emodin, aloetic acid, alovin and anthracine polysaccharides

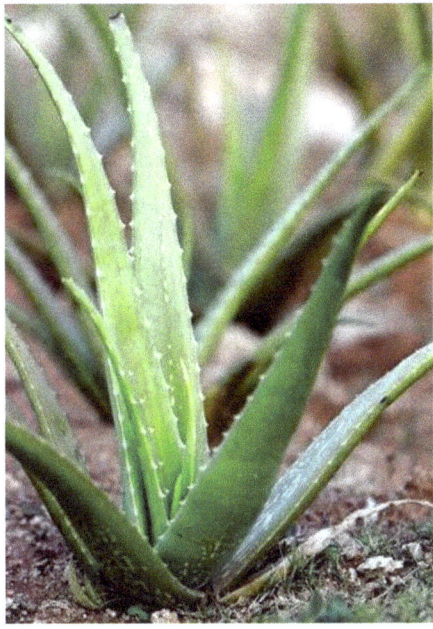
Aloes

(glucomannans and polymannose), and lupeol. (88, 129, 130)
Pharmacological Activity: Antibacterial effects of compounds in *A. vera* inclusive of anthraquinones, saponins and steroids have been reported. Polysaccharides from *A. vera* gel has comparable antitussive activity to dropropizine. (88, 129)

Kalanchoe pinnata (Lam.) Pers. [DC005]
Wonder of the World
Family: Crassulaceae
Local Preparation: Wash leaf and eat or boil into a tea to help cough. (1)
Bioactive Chemical Profile: Reducing sugars, terpenoids, steroids, cardiac glycosides, tannins, phlobatannins, saponins, anthraquinone, flavonosides, flavonoids and resins. (131)

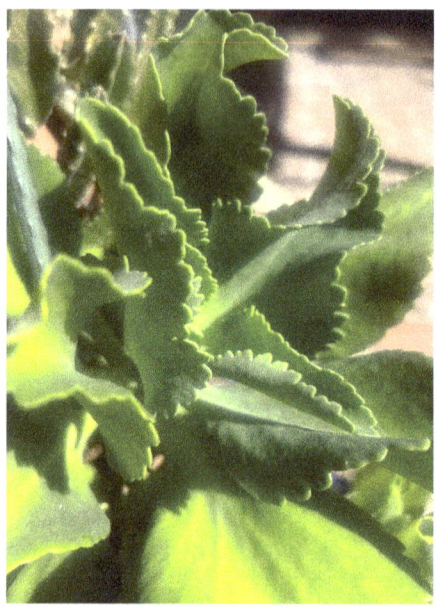
Wonder of the World

Marrubium vulgare L.
Horehound
Family: Lamiaceae
Local Preparation: Steeped in hot water (hot infusion) for coughs. (1)
Bioactive Chemical Profile: Marrubiin, marrbiol, murrubenol, alkaloids, sesquiterpene, tannin, saponins and resin. (133)
Pharmacological Activity: The methanol extract of *M. vulgare* showed significant antimicrobial activities against E*scherichia coli, Bacillus subtilis, Staphylococcus aureus, Staphylococcus epidermidis, Pseudomonas aeruginosa, Proteus vulgaris* and *Candida albicans*. (252)

Pharmacological Activity: The n-hexane soluble fraction of an ethanolic extract of the *K. pinnata* leaves showed antimicrobial activity by zones of inhibition (in parenthesis) against selected microorganisms with the highest bioactivity against *Staphylococcus aureus* (12mm), *Klebsiella pneumonia* (11mm) and *Salmonella typhi* (8mm). The ethyl acetate soluble fraction showed mild antimicrobial activity against *Escherichia coli* (6mm), *Staphylococcus aureus* (7mm) and *Salmonella typhi* (7mm). Both extracts were tested at a concentration of 10 mg/ml using the paper disc technique described by Bauer-Kirby. (131, 132)

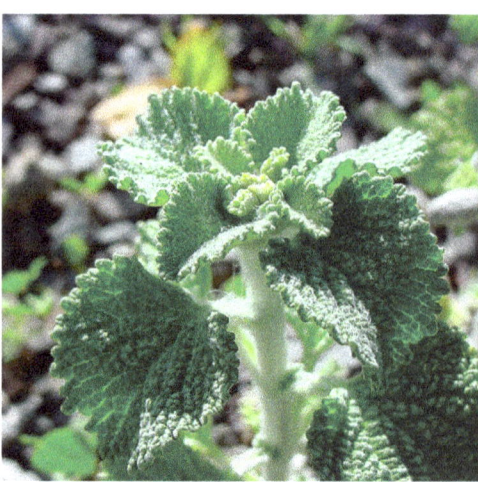
Horebound

Azadirachta indica A. Juss.
Neem
Family: Meliaceae
Local Preparation: A decoction of the leaves to help coughs. (1)
Bioactive Chemical Profile: Nimbin, nimbidin (antibacterial), quercetin,

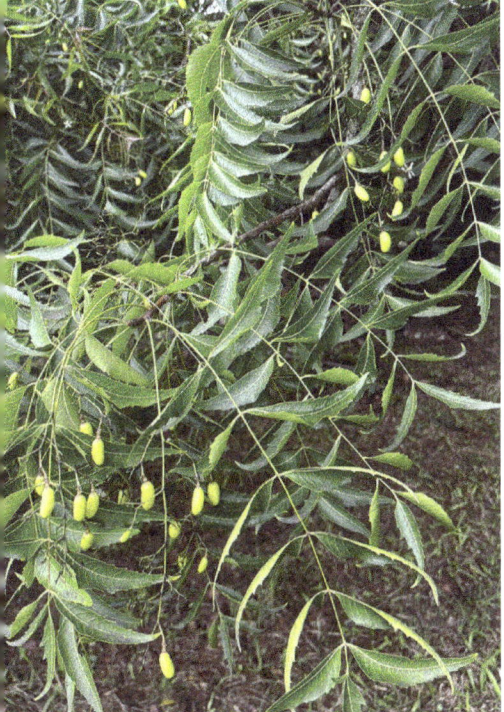

Neem

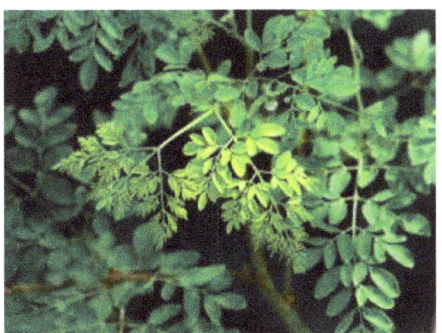

Moringa

Moringa oleifera Lam.
Moringa
Family: Moringaceae
Local Preparation: Seeds chewed to help cough. (1)
Bioactive Chemical Profile:
The aqueous and hydro-alcoholic extracts of the seeds contain methionine, cysteine, 4-(alpha-L- rhamnopyranosyloxy) benzylglucosinolate, Moringine, benzylglucosinolate, niazimicin and niazarin. (253)
Pharmacological Activity: The plant shows *in vitro* activity against bacteria, yeast, dermatophytes and helminths by the disc diffusion method. The aqueous extract of the fresh leaves and the seeds inhibit the growth of *Pseudomonas aeruginosa* and *Staphylococcus aureu*s. (253)

limonoids, terpenoids, sterols, fatty acids, coumarins, azadiradione, hydrocarbons, sulphur containing compounds and phenolics. (34, 35)
Pharmacological Activity: Neem oil has been shown to inhibit many strains of pathogenic bacteria such as *Staphylococcus aureus* in clinical trials. Oil from the leaves, seed and bark possesses a wide spectrum of antibacterial action against Gram-negative and Gram-positive microorganisms such as *Mycobacterium tuberculosis* and streptomycin resistant strains. Nimbidin has antibacterial properties. (34, 35)

Pimenta racemosa (Mill.) J.W. Moore [DC018]
Bay Leaf
Family: Myrtaceae
Local Preparation: A decoction of the leaves to help sinusitis. (1)

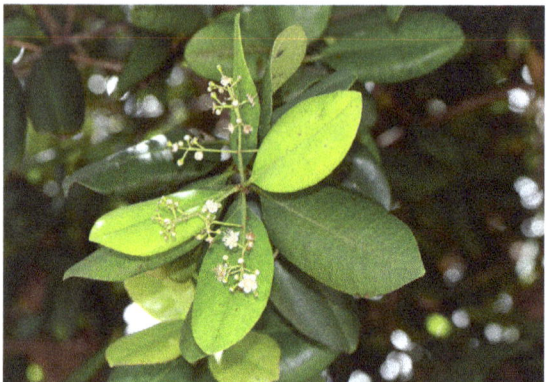
Bay Leaf

Bioactive Chemical Profile: Terpenoids, steroids, saponins, phenolic nuclei, glycosides, tannins, and quinines. 1,8-cineole, linalool and myrcene were noted as major constituents in the essential oils of the flower. (62, 116)

Pharmacological Activity: Antimicrobial effects of the essential oils of the flowers have been reported against *Bacillus subtilis, Geotrichum candidum, Staphylococcus aureus* and *Penicillium italicum* with minimum inhibitory concentrations ranging from 0.49–6.22 μg/ml. These effects were noted to be comparable to ampicillin and amphotericin B antibiotic standards. (116)

Psidium guajava L.
Guava
Family: Myrtaceae
Local Preparation: Fruit eaten to help a sore throat. (1)
Bioactive Chemical Profile: Catechins and gallic acid. (134)

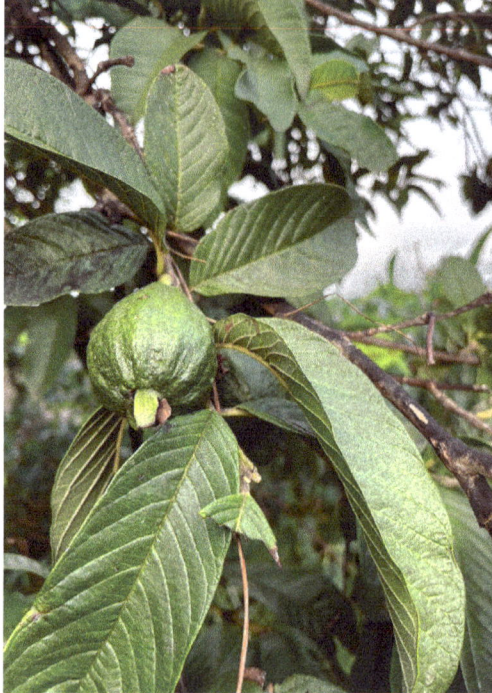
Guava

Pharmacological Activity: The antimicrobial effects of aqueous and acetone-water extracts of *Psidium guajava* were reported as very effective against the Gram-positive bacterium *Staphylococcus epidermidis* and the Gram-negative bacterium *Shigella flexneri* on evaluation of the minimum inhibitory concentration values. (134)

Cymbopogon citratus (DC.) Stapf [DC0001]
Lemongrass
Family: Poaceae
Local Preparation: Hot infusion of the leaves for cough and sinusitis. (1)

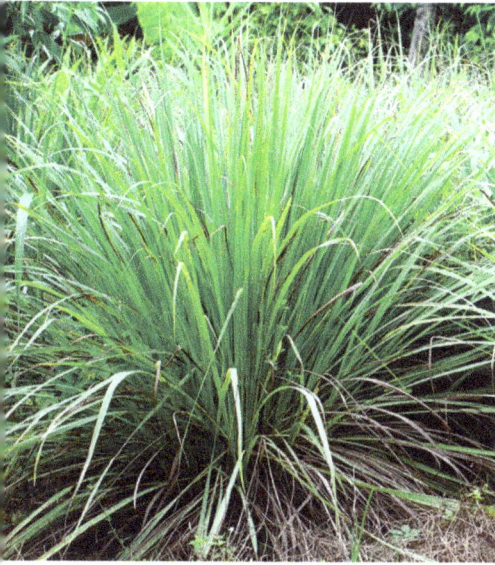
Lemongrass

Bioactive Chemical Profile: Essential oils inclusive of geranial (citral α), neral (citral β) and citronellal are present along with flavonoids and phenolic compounds such as quercetin, kaempferol and tannic acid. (135)

Pharmacological Activity: The essential oils of *C. citratus* showed greatest antibacterial activity, followed by the plant's methanolic extract. The essential oil extract of *C. citratus* also exhibited better antibacterial activity in Gram-positive bacteria than in Gram-negative bacteria, with the exception of *Pseudomonas aeruginosa* which showed a high susceptibility towards the methanolic extract. Bacterial isolates tested were methicillin-resistant Staphylococcus aureus (MRSA), methicillin-susceptible *Staphylococcus aureus* (MSSA), methicillin-resistant *Staphylococcus epidermidis* (MRSE), *Enterococcus faecalis, Staphylococcus aureus, Staphylococcus epidermidis* and gram-negative bacteria *(Acinetobacter baummanii, Citrobacter freundii, Enterobacter cloacae, Escherichia coli, Klebsiella pneumoniae, Proteus mirabilis, Proteus vulgaris* and *Pseudomonas aeruginosa*). Kaempferol and quercetin have been shown to suppress mucus production in airways. (135, 136)

Morinda citrifolia L
Noni, Dog dumpling, Monkey dumpling, Forbidden fruit, Wild pine (3)
Family: Rubiaceae
Local Preparation: Extraction of the fruit to gargle for sore throats. An application of the leaf and fruit to treat abscesses.

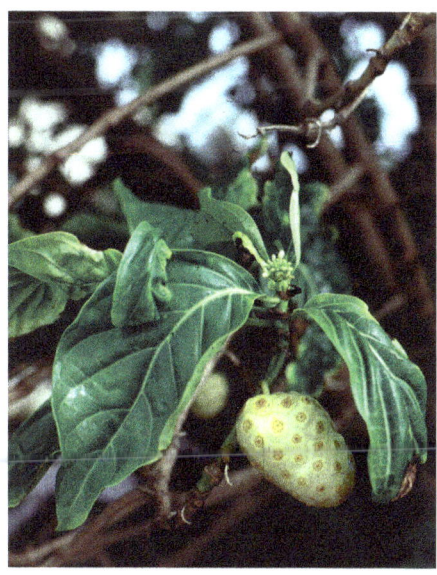
Noni, Dog dumpling, Monkey dumpling, Forbidden fruit, Wild pine

Bioactive Chemical Profile: The leaves have several iridoids, flavonol glycosides and triterpenes. Both leaves and seeds have quinones and coumarins which are associated with antimicrobial effects. Polysaccharides, fatty acid glycosides, iridoids, anthraquinones, coumarins, flavonoids, lignans, phytosterols, carotinoids, monoterpenes, short chain fatty acids and fatty acid esters are more associated with the fruit. (137, 138)

Pharmacological Activity: The antimicrobial activity of the alcoholic, hexanoic, chloroform and ethyl acetate extracts from the leaves and seeds of *M. citrifolia* L. (noni) were reported against *Escherichia coli* and *Staphylococcus aureus* using the Bauer-Kirby method. The seed extract of the plant has reported the best antibacterial activity. (138, 139)

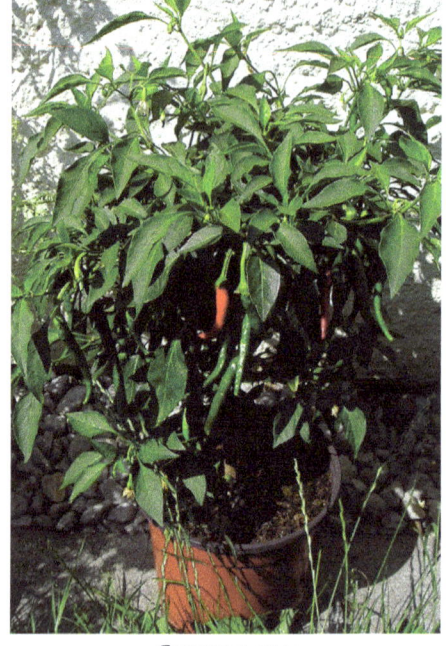

Cayenne pepper

Capsicum annuum L.
Cayenne pepper
Family: Solanaceae
Local Preparation: Extract used for sinusitis. (1)
Bioactive Chemical Profile: Capsaicin, luteolin and apigenin. (140)
Pharmacological Activity: A fraction of *C. anuum* derived from reverse-phase HPLC displayed significant antimicrobial activity against *Listeria monocytogenes, Escherichia coli* and *Salmonella enterica* compared to control samples. Mass spectra analysis revealed that fractions contained compounds belonging to a group of *C. annuum-specific* compounds known as capsianosides. (141, 142)

Curcuma longa L.
Turmeric
Family: Zingiberaceae
Local Preparation: Decoction or hot infusion of the rhizome for sinusitis. (2)

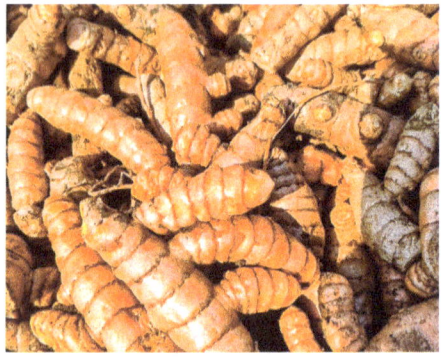

Turmeric

Bioactive Chemical Profile: Curcumin. (126)
Pharmacological Activity: Antimicrobial effects have been reported prior in this text (127, 128) Curcumin has been shown to improve nasal airflow, alleviate inflammation, and provided beneficial effects in experimentally induced sinusitis. (143, 144)

Zingiber officinale Roscoe
Ginger
Family: Zingiberaceae
Local Preparation: Decoction of rhizome for sinusitis. (1) Hot infusion of grated or whole rhizomes to help dyspnea. (1)
Bioactive Chemical Profile: Gingerol, shogaol and decanal. (145)

Pharmacological Activity: The ethanolic extract of ginger exhibited potent antibacterial activities against respiratory tract pathogens including *Staphylococcus aureus, Streptococcus pyogenes & Streptococcus pneumoniae.* The minimum inhibitory concentrations of the ginger extract ranged from 0.0003 µg/ml to 0.7 µg/ml. Anti-inflammatory properties have also been reported. (145, 146)

VIRAL INFECTION – COLD, INFLUENZA & CHICKEN POX VIRUS

Achyranthes aspera L. var aspera
Hug-Me-Close
Family: Amaranthacae
Local Preparation: Hot infusion of the leaves for influenza.

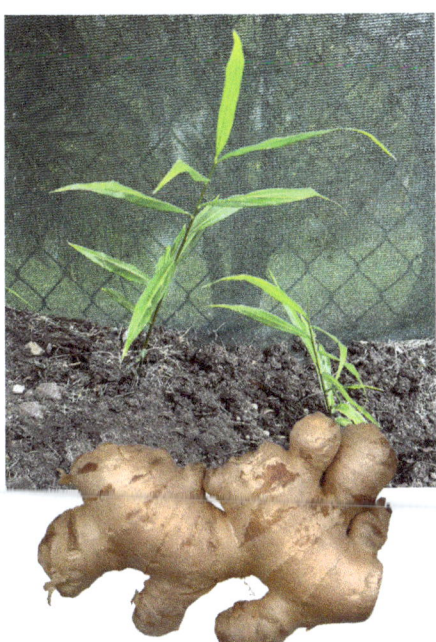

Ginger

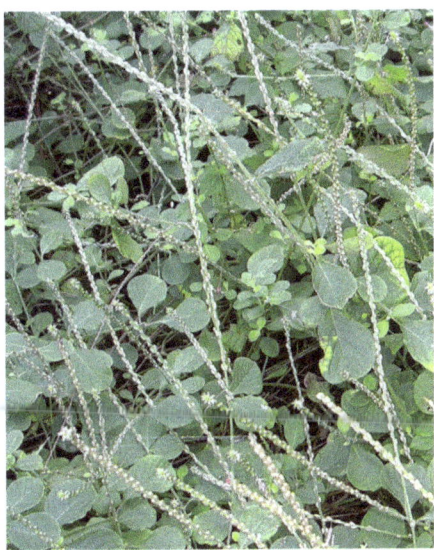

Hug-Me-Close

Bioactive Chemical Profile: Fatty acids (oleanolic acid), flavonoids, phenols and acylquinic acids. (147)
Pharmacological Activity: The methanolic extract of *Achyranthes aspera* possessed antiviral activity against the Herpes simplex virus (HSV) with a potency (EC_{50}) of 64.4µg/ml for HSV-1 and 72.8µg/ml for HSV-2). Also, oleanolic acid exhibited anti-herpes viral activity against both HSV-1 and HSV-2 with a potency (EC_{50}) of 6.8µg/ml and 7.8µg/ml respectively. (148)

Aloe vera (L.) Burm.f. [DC009]
Aloes
Family: Asphodelaceae
Local Preparation: Leaves blended and squeezed. (1)
Bioactive Chemical Profile: Quercetin, catechin, kaempferol and anthraquinones. (149, 150)
Pharmacological Activity: The ethanolic extract of *A. vera* significantly reduces the viral replication of green fluorescent protein-labeled influenza A virus in Madin-Darby canine kidney (MDCK) cells. (149, 150)

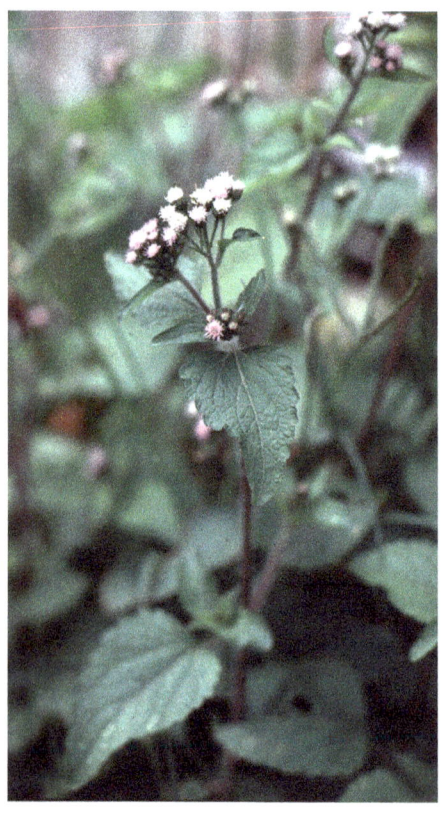

Wild Ageratum

Ageratum conyzoides L.
Wild Ageratum
Family: Asteraceae
Local Preparation: A hot infusion of the plant for colds.
Bioactive Chemical Profile: Alkaloids, coumarins, flavonoids, chromenes, benzofurans, sterols and terpenoids. (89)
Pharmacological Activity: An extract of *Ageratum conyzoides* showed potent antiviral activity with IC_{50} of 0.208 µg/mL and 0.006 µg/mL against two serotypes of echoviruses E7 and E19 respectively. (151)

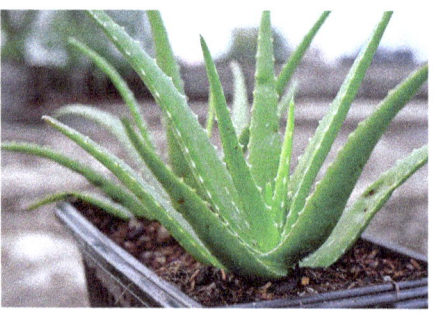

Aloe vera

Ambrosia hispida Pursh
Wild Geranium, Seaside Geranium
Family: Asteraceae
Local Preparation: A hot infusion of the leaves for colds.
Bioactive Chemical Profile: Leaf extract has 84 essential oils with major constituents, borneol (19.4%) and spathulenol (11.8%). (48)

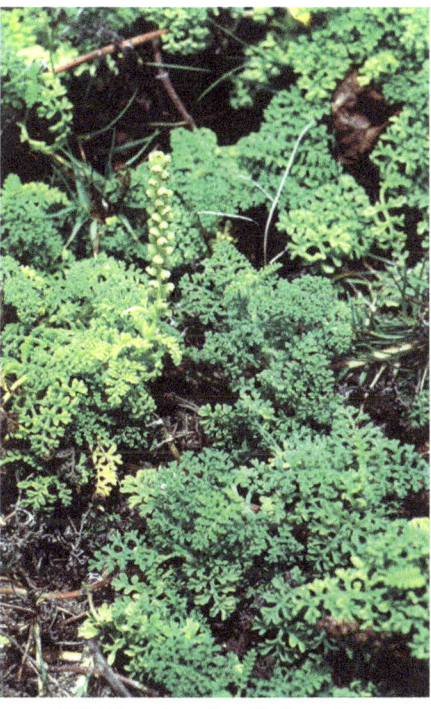

Wild Geranium, Seaside Geranium

Pharmacological Activity: A novel series of borneol derivatives containing different heterocyclic fragments showed antiviral effects with IC_{50} ranging from 3.2 and > 1886.8 µM against the influenza virus A/Puerto Rico/8/34 (H1N1) in MDCK cells. (152)

Bidens alba (L.) var. *radiata* DC. (Sch. Bip.) Ballard
Duppy Needles, Monkey Needles, Spanish Needles (1)
Family: Asteraceae
Local Preparation: A hot infusion of the leaves for colds.
Bioactive Chemical Profile: Flavonoids, polyacetylenic compounds (cytopiloyne) and tannins have been found in related species *B. Pilosa*. (23, 47)
Pharmacological Activity: A hot-water extract of *B. pilosa* significantly inhibited the replication of Herpes simplex virus (HSV) at a concentration of 100 µg/ml (11.9% for HSV-1 and 19.2% for HSV-2. (153)

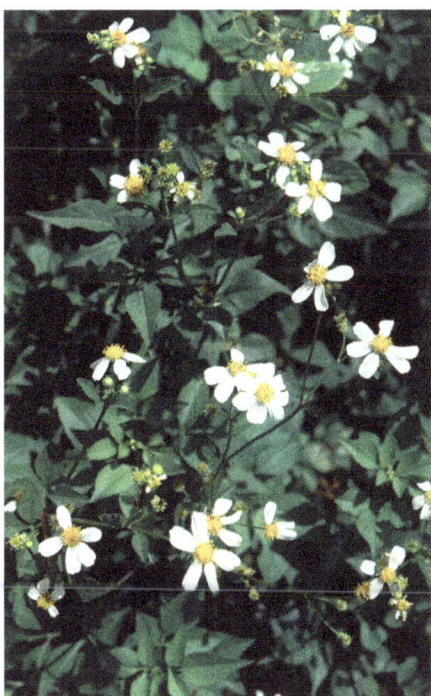

Duppy Needles, Monkey Needles, Spanish Needles

Borrichia arborescens (L.) DC
Seabush
Family: Asteraceae
Local Preparation: Decoction of the leaves.

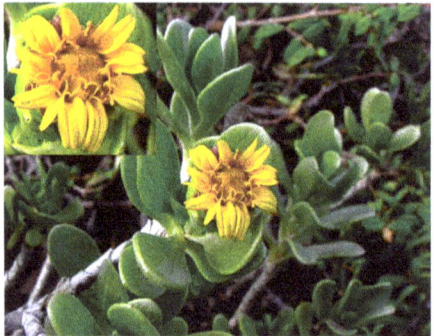
Seabush

Bioactive Chemical Profile: No phytochemical profile of plant has been published to date.
Pharmacological Activity: No antiviral activity has been reported to date.

Eclipta prostrata (L.) L
Conga Lala (1)
Family: Asteraceae
Local Preparation: Decoction or hot infusion of the leaves and other plant parts.
Bioactive Chemical Profile: Alkenynes, alkaloids, cardiac glycosides, flavonoids, coumestans, lipids, polyacetylene, steroids, saponins, steroidal alkaloids, phytosterol and triterpenes. (154)
Pharmacological Activity: The coumestans are reported as the most common bioactive compounds in the plant and contribute to the reported

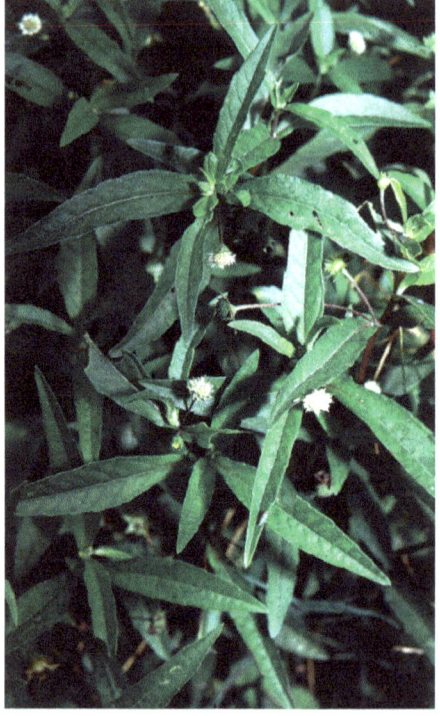
Conga Lala

antiviral effects against the Human immunodeficiency virus (HIV). (154)

Eupatorium odoratum L
Jack-in-the-Bush
Family: Asteraceae
Local Preparation: Decoction of the leaves for colds and influenza.
Bioactive Chemical Profile: Phytosterols, triterpenes, alkaloids, flavonoids, tannins, diterpenes, and saponins, glycosides, lactones and diterpenes. (155)
Pharmacological Activity: The anti-viral activity of the extracts of the plant has not been appropriately investigated. The antioxidant and

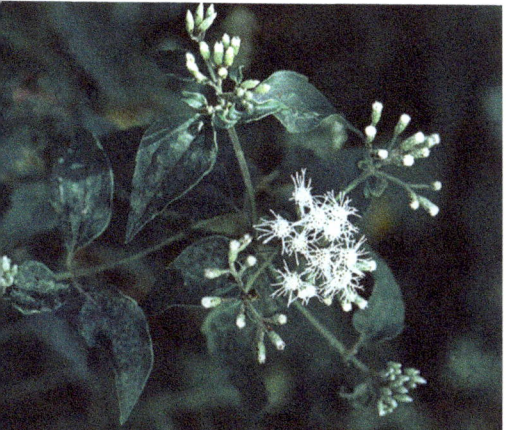

Jack-in-the-Bush

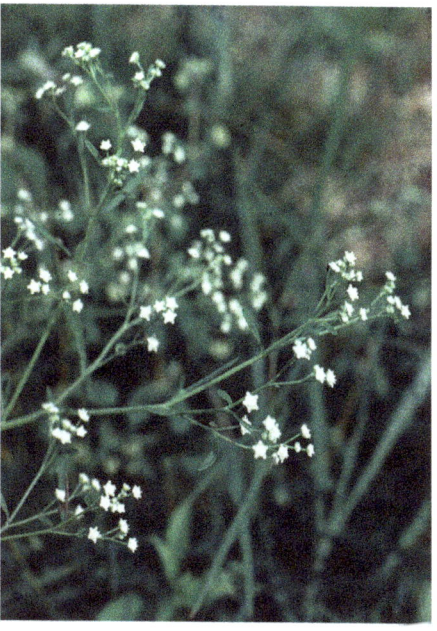

Whitehead Bush

anti-inflammatory effects of the plant's phytochemicals may be beneficial in improving symptoms associated with viral infections. (254)

Parthenium hysterophorus L
Whitehead Bush
Family: Asteraceae
Local Preparation: A hot infusion of the leaves for colds.
Bioactive Chemical Profile:
Apigenin, borneoil, camphor, canin, carminarone, coronopilin, luteolin, parthenin, parthenolide, pathenolide, a-pinene, reynosin, santamarin, santin, tetraneurin E, caffeic, vanllic, ferulic, chlorogenic and anisic acids. (156)
Pharmacological Activity:
Parthenolide, a sesquiterpene lactone, exerts anti-Herpes simplex virus-1 (HSV-1) activity with a potency (EC_{50}) of 0.3 μg/ml by the Plaque Reduction Assay method. It impairs cell viability, which consequently interferes with the efficient infection and production of new viral particles. (157)

Pluchea carolinensis (Jacq.) G. Don
Cure-for-All
Family: Asteraceae
Local Preparation: Decoction of the leaves for colds and influenza.
Bioactive Chemical Profile:
Sesquiterpenoids and flavonoids are the main constituents of the plant. (158)
Pharmacological Activity: A related species, *P. indica* showed antiviral effects against Human immunodeficiency virus type 1 (HIV-1) with antiviral selectivity index of 94 determined by 50% cytotoxic concentration /50% effective antiviral concentration. (159)

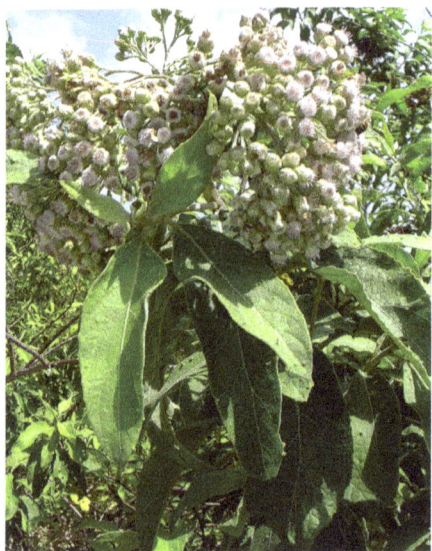
Cure-for-All

Syndrella nodiflora (L.) Gaertn
Porter Bush
Family: Asteraceae
Local Preparation: A hot infusion or decoction is used for colds.
Bioactive Chemical Profile: Quinic acids (chlorogenic and neochlorogenic). (160, 161)

Pharmacological Activity: The hydro-ethanolic extract of *S. nodiflora* contains phenolic compounds which may be responsible for the antioxidant properties at a concentration of 0.1–3.0 mg/ml. (160, 161) These antioxidant effects improve symptoms associated with viral infections.

Guilandina bonduc L.
Horsenicker
Family: Caesalpiniaceae
Local Preparation: A hot infusion of the leaves for colds.
Bioactive Chemical Profile: Flavonoids, tannins, alkaloids, phytosterols, saponins, coumarins, triterpenoids, furano- cassane-diterpenes, nor-cassane diterpenes and neo-cassane diterpenes. (162, 163)
Pharmacological Activity: The ethanolic extract of the root and stem of *Guilandina bonduc* exhibited activity against the Vaccinia virus. (163)

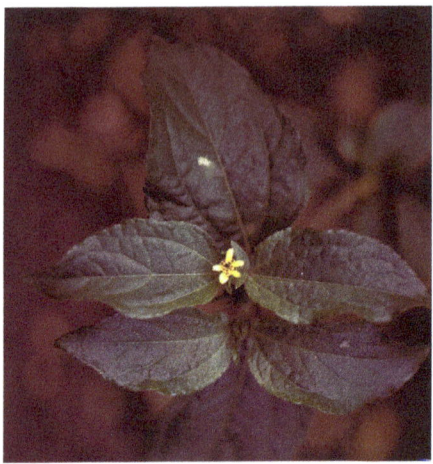
Porter Bush

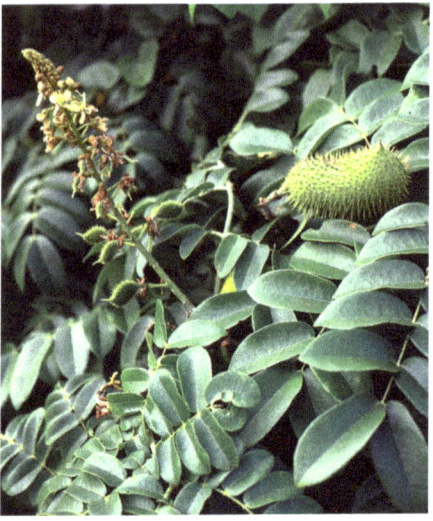
Horsenicker

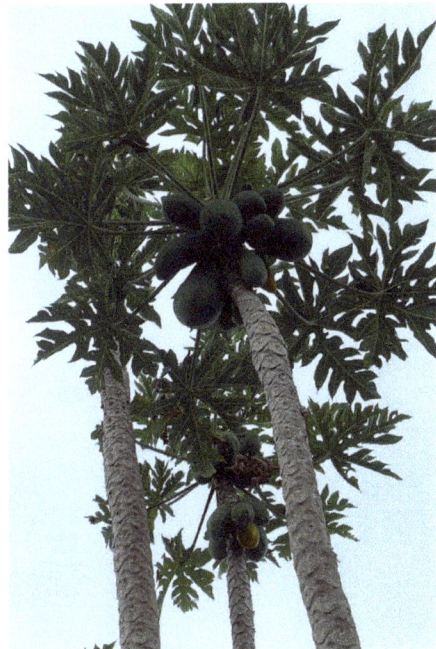

Pawpaw, Papaya

Carica papaya L. [DC011]
Pawpaw, Papaya
Family: Caricaceae
Local Preparation: Leaves boiled. (1)
Bioactive Chemical Profile: Carpaine, dehydrocarpaine I and II, cardenolide, p-coumaric acid, chlorogenic acid, caricaxanthin, violaxanthin and zeaxanthin. (164)
Pharmacological Activity:
Potential anti-viral activity has been demonstrated using an *in silico* docking method with carpaine, dehydrocarpaine I and II, cardenolide, p-coumaric acid, chlorogenic acid, caricaxanthin, violaxanthin and zeaxanthin against a number of viruses e.g., Dengue, Influenza A and the Chikungunya virus. (164)

Kalanchoe pinnata (Lam.) Pers. [DC005]
Wonder of the World
Family: Crassulaceae
Local Preparation: Blend and squeeze leaves or a decoction of the dried leaves.
Bioactive Chemical Profile:
Flavonoids, phenols, bufadienolides and scaphopetalone. (165)
Pharmacological Activity: Two compounds isolated from *K. pinnata*, KPB-100 and KPB-200, inhibited Human alpha-herpes virus 2 (HSV-2) at IC_{50} values of 2.5 and 2.9 µg/ml respectively and the Vaccinia virus (VACV) at IC_{50} values of 3.1 and 7.4 µg/mL respectively in plaque reduction assays. (165)

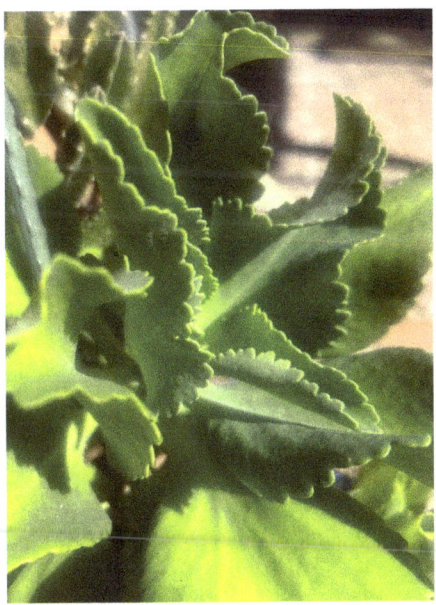

Wonder of the World

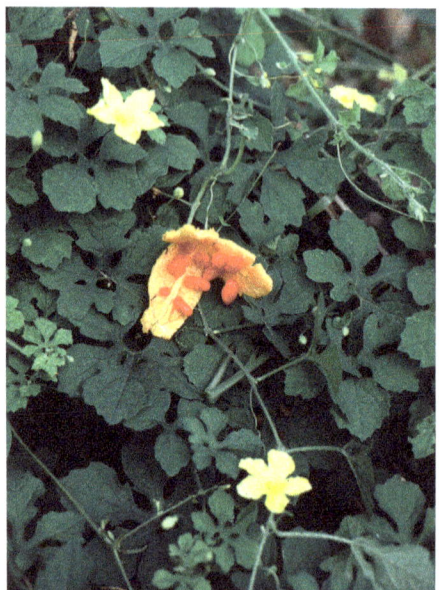

Cerasee

Momordica charantia L. [DC002]
Cerasee
Family: Cucurbitaceae
Local Preparation: Decoction of the leaves and stem into a tea. (1, 2)
Bioactive Chemical Profile:
Triterpenoids, saponins, polypeptides, flavonoids, alkaloids, sterols, Kuguacin C & E, MAP30, MRK29 and momordicin. (166)
Pharmacological Activity: Ethanolic extracts from leaves and stems of *M. charantia* highly inhibit Herpes simplex virus – 1 (HSV-1) and Sindbis virus (SINV). Kuguacin C and Kuguacin E isolated from the root of *M. charantia* showed moderate antiviral activity against Human immunodeficiency virus – 1 (HIV-1) with a potency (EC_{50}) of 8.45 and 25.62 µg/mL respectively. (166, 167)

Croton flavens L.
Yellow Balsam, Seaside Sage (1)
Family: Euphorbiacae
Local Preparation: A hot infusion of the sap with sugar or syrup for colds and coughs.
Bioactive Chemical Profile:
Terpenoids (diterpenoids), mono and sesquiterpenoids, and sometimes, shikimate-derived compounds, alkaloids, phenolic compounds (flavonoids, lignoids and proanthocyanidins) predominate. (168)

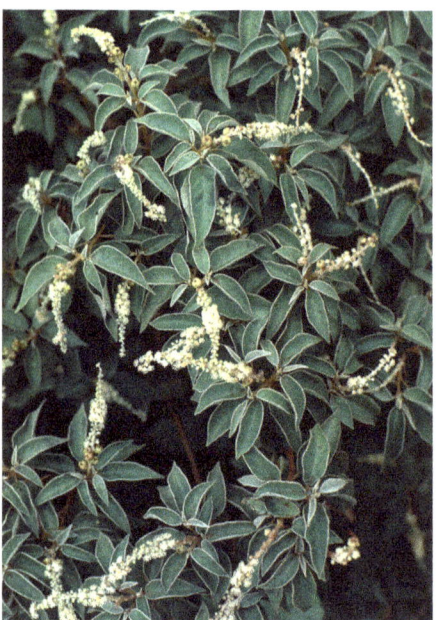

Yellow Balsam, Seaside Sage

Pharmacological Activity:
SP-303, a large proanthocyanidin oligomer isolated from the latex of the plant species *Croton lechleri* has demonstrated broad activity against a variety of DNA and RNA viruses. (168, 169)

Phyllanthus epiphyllanthus L.
Monkey Spoon, Herringbone (1)
Family: Euphorbiacae
Local Preparation: Chew and spit out the leaves to relieve colds and coughs.
Bioactive Chemical Profile:
Terpenoids, phenylpropanoids, tannins, flavonoids, sterols, alkaloids and phenolic compounds can be found in the genus Phyllanthus. (170)

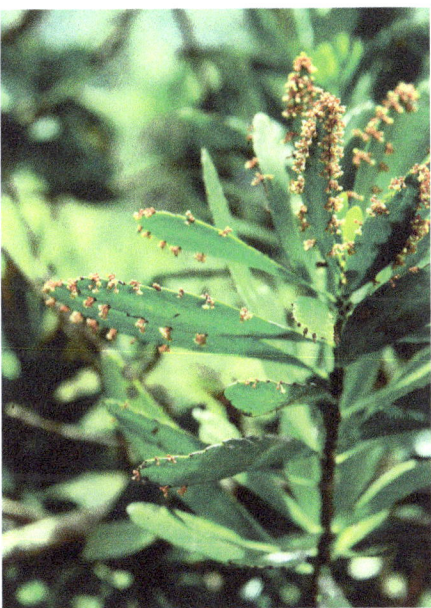

Monkey Spoon, Herringbone

Pharmacological Activity: Various Phyllanthus plants were reported to have strong antiviral potential against Human immunodeficiency virus (HIV), Hepatitis C, Herpes simplex virus and Cytomegalovirus (HCMV). The aqueous extract of *P. emblica* reduced viral load of HIV significantly at the dose of 400 µg/ml. Aqueous extract of *P. orbicularis* revealed inhibition activity against the replication of HCMV, HSV-1, and HSV-2 as well as Bovine herpesvirus 1 (BHV-1) with potencies (EC_{50}) of 57.7, 28.8, 25.7, and 21.27 µg/mL, respectively. (170)

Phyllanthus amarus Schum.
Seed-Under-Leaf
Family: Euphorbiacae
Local Preparation: Decoction of the leaves, seeds and stems.
Bioactive Chemical Profile:
Terpenoids, phenylpropanoids, tannins, flavonoids, sterols, alkaloids and phenolic compounds can be found in the genus Phyllanthus. (170)
Pharmacological Activity: Various Phyllanthus plants were reported to have strong antiviral potential against Human immunodeficiency virus (HIV), Hepatitis C (HCV), Herpes simplex virus and Cytomegalovirus (HCMV). (170–172).

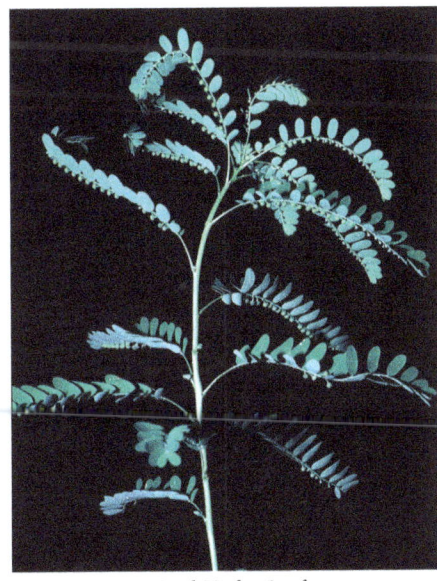

Seed-Under-Leaf

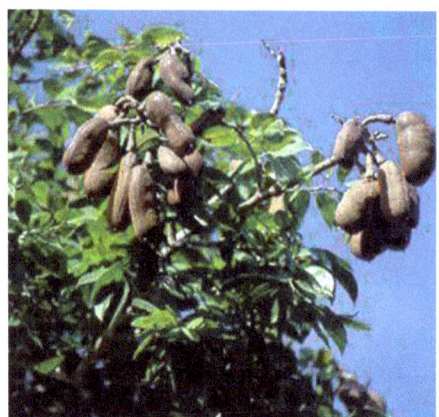

Locust Tree, Stinking Toe Tree

Hymenaea courbaril L.
Locust Tree, Stinking Toe Tree
Family: Fabaceae
Local Preparation: Decoction of the bark for respiratory ailments.
Bioactive Chemical Profile: Saponins, flavonoids, tannins (astilbin), coumarins and terpenes found in the leaf extracts that showed antiviral activity. (173, 174)
Pharmacological Activity: A study demonstrated potent antioxidant properties, myorelaxant and anti-inflammatory activities of an ethanol crude extract of the stem bark. The ethanolic crude extract of the leaves exhibited strong *in vitro* activity against Rotavirus at a concentration range of 50–500 μg/ml. No amplification of genetic material was observed from the Rotavirus. (173, 174)

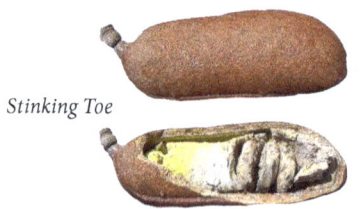

Stinking Toe

Senna occidentalis (L.) Link
Stinking Bush (1)
Family: Fabaceae
Local Preparation: A hot infusion of the leaves for colds.
Bioactive Chemical Profile: Saponins, sterols, flavonoids, resins, alkaloids, terpenes, anthraquinones, glycoside and balsam. (175, 176)

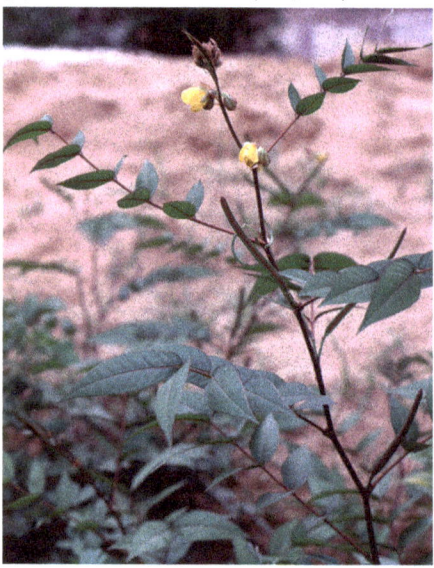

Stinking bush

Pharmacological Activity: Saponins from the plant have been reported to have antiviral effects. (176)

Leonotis nepetifolia (L.) Ait. F.
Lion Head, Man Piabba, Ball Bush, Hot Bush
Family: Lamiaceae
Local Preparation: A hot infusion of the leaves for colds.
Bioactive Chemical Profile: Labdane diterpenoids, coumarins, bis-spirolabdane diterpenes, flavonoids,

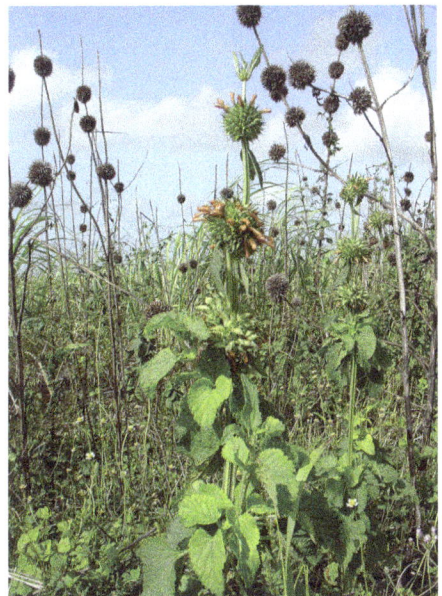

Lion Head, Man Piabba, Bull Bush, Hot Bush

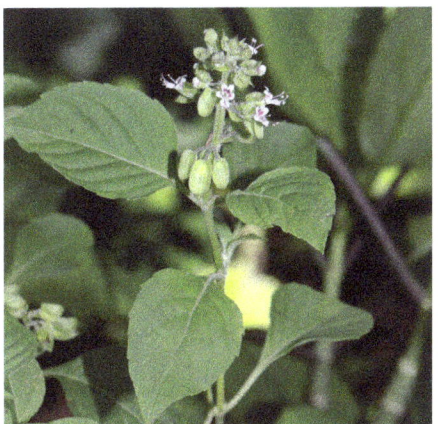

Duppy Basil, Mosquito Bush

fatty esters, iridoils, iridoid glycosides, phenylethanoids, allenic acid and coumarins. (177, 178)

Pharmacological Activity: Antiviral effects of the methanolic, ethanolic and hexane extracts of the leaves of *L. nepetofolia* have been reported. (177)

Ocimum campechianum Miller
Duppy Basil, Mosquito Bush
Family: Lamiaceae
Local Preparation: A hot infusion of the leaves.
Bioactive Chemical Profile:
Eugenol, methyl eugenol, carvacrol, sesquiterpine, apigenin, luteolin and ursolic acid. (179)
Pharmacological Activity: Ursolic acid has shown antiviral effects against Herpes simplex virus-1 (HSV-1), Adenovirus-8 (ADV-8), Coxsackievirus B1 (CVB1) and Enterovirus 71 with potency and selectivity indices (in parenthesis) of 6.6 mg/l (15.2), 4.2 mg/l (23.8) 0.4 mg/L (251.3) and 0.5 mg/l (201) respectively. (180)

Malachra alceifolia Jacq.
Wild Okra
Family: Malvaceae
Local Preparation: A hot infusion of the leaves for colds and cough.

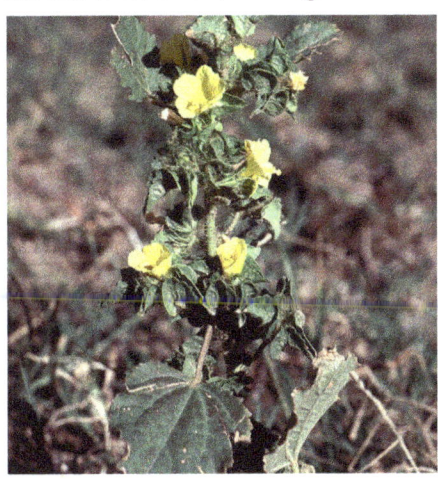

Wild Okra

Bioactive Chemical Profile: The genus *Malachra* contains flavonoids; compounds of phenolic acids, phytosterol; fatty acid derivatives; alkaloids, tannins and dipeptide in the leaves, stems, flowers, and root, fresh or dried. (255)

Pharmacological Activity: The antiviral effects of the plant have not been validated in the literature to date.

Sida rhombifolia L.
Arrow Leaf
Family: Malvaceae
Local Preparation: A decoction of the plant (leaves and aerial parts).
Bioactive Chemical Profile: Coumarins (scoparone). (60)
Pharmacological Activity: Coumarins (e.g., scoparone found in *S. rhombifolia*) are emerging as potent anti-viral agents, exhibiting antiviral activity against Human immunodeficiency virus (HIV), Hepatitis C (HCV), Infuenza virus and others. In one study, a coumarin derivative, eleutheroside B1, showed a wide spectrum of anti-human influenza virus effect with IC_{50} value of 64–125µg/ml *in vitro*. (60, 181, 182)

Thespesia populnea (L.) Sol. Ex Correa
Anodyne, Mahoe (1)
Family: Malvaceae
Local Preparation: A hot infusion of the leaves for colds.
Bioactive Chemical Profile: Flavonoids, gallic acid and catechin. (183, 184)
Pharmacological Activity: A flavonoid-rich extract demonstrated significant antiviral activities against vesicular stomatitis, coxsackie, and respiratory syncytical viruses at a potency (EC_{50}) of 20 µg/ml. (183)

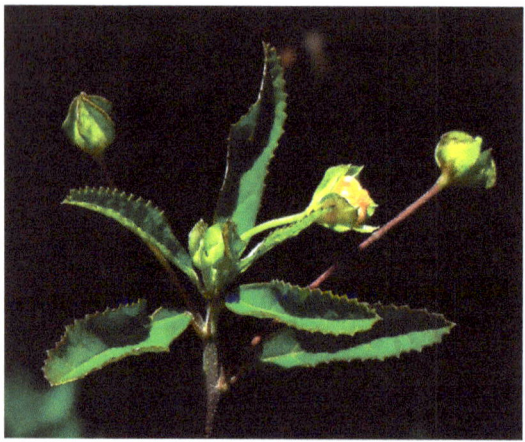
Arrow leaf

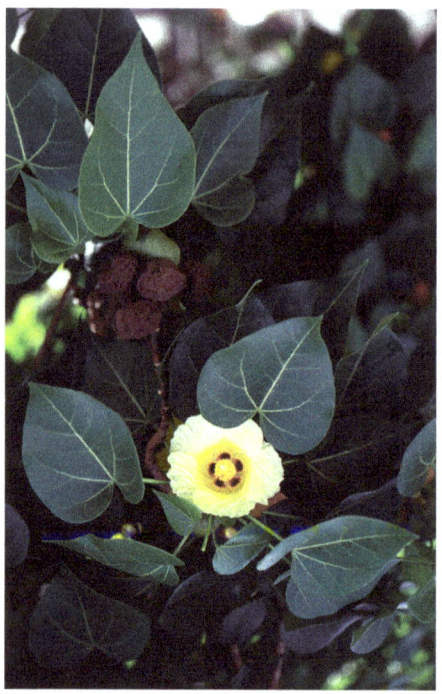
Anodyne, Mahoe

Urena lobata L. (30)
Caesarweed; Congo jute
Family: Malvaceae
Local Preparation: A hot infusion or decoction of the leaves or flowers for colds and influenza.
Bioactive Chemical Profile:
Kaempferol glycosides, quercetin and imperatorin. (185)
Pharmacological Activity:
Significant antiviral activities of the identified phytochemicals have been reported previously (e.g., inhibition

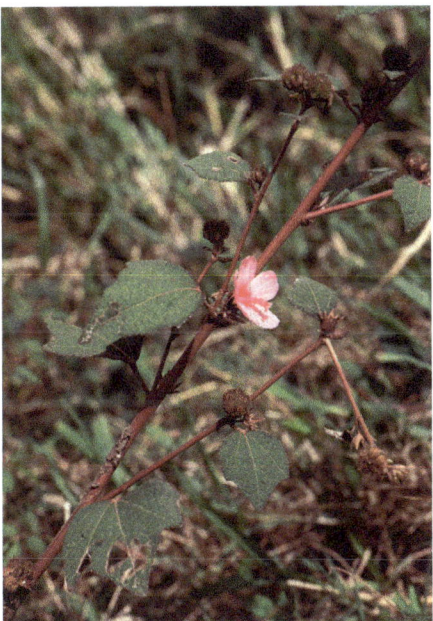

Caesarweed; Congo jute

of viral replication and release). Kaempferol, kaempferol glycosides, and acylated kaempferol glucoside derivatives can block the 3a channel of the severe acute respiratory syndrome (SARS) coronavirus. The most effective one was the glycoside juglanin (carrying an arabinose residue) with an IC_{50} value of 2.3 μM. (186, 187)

Cymbopogon citratus (DC.) Stapf [DC001]
Lemongrass
Family: Poaceae
Local Preparation: A hot Infusion of the leaves.
Bioactive Chemical Profile: The chemical composition of the essential oil of *Cymbopogon citratus* includes hydrocarbon terpenes, alcohols, ketones, esters and mainly aldehydes. Citral is the acyclic monoterpene aldehyde that exists in the essential oils. These compounds may be limited in the aqueaous extract. (256)
Pharmacological Activity: An extract of the closely related species, *Cymbopogon nardus,* obtained with 80% ethanol (CN80) displayed potential activity against Human mastadenovirus serotype 5 (HAdV-5), at a concentration of 75 μg/ml. (188)

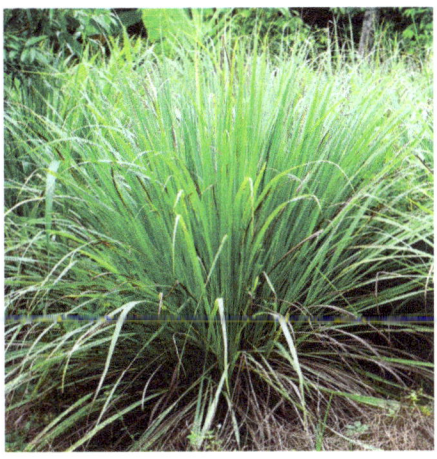

Lemongrass

Hedyotis verticillata (L.) Lam.
Buttonweed
Family: Rubiaceae
Local Preparation: A hot infusion of the leaves for colds.
Bioactive Chemical Profile: Rutin and chlorogenic acid. (189)
Pharmacological Activity: Chlorogenic acid is effective in combatting viral upper respiratory tract infections. It showed inhibitory activity against the novel influenzas A/PuertoRico/8/1934 (H1N1) and A/Beijing/32/92 (H3N2) with potencies (EC_{50}) of 44.87 µM and 62.33 µM respectively. These effects were also observed in oseltamivir-resistant strains. It also exhibited anti-tussive and expectorant effects, as well as alleviating acute airway inflammation. (190, 191)

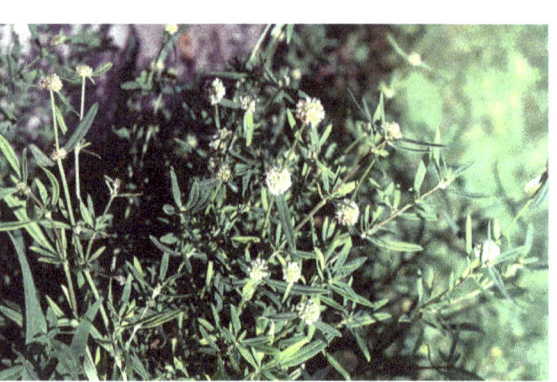

Buttonweed

Psychotria nervosa Sw.
St. John's Bush
Family: Rubiaceae
Local Preparation: Decoction of the leaves for colds. Leaves also used in a mixed bush tea for colds.
Bioactive Chemical Profile: The genus Psychotria's phytochemical profile includes alkaloids (indole, monoterpene indole, quinoline and isoquinoline), flavonoids, coumarins, terpenoids and cyclic peptides. (119)
Pharmacological Activity: Ementine, an alkaloid from the Psychotria species inhibited Human immunodeficiency virus (HIV) replication by interfering with reverse transcriptase activity. The ethanolic extract from *P. serpens* significantly suppressed Herpes simplex virus type 1 (HSP-1). (119)

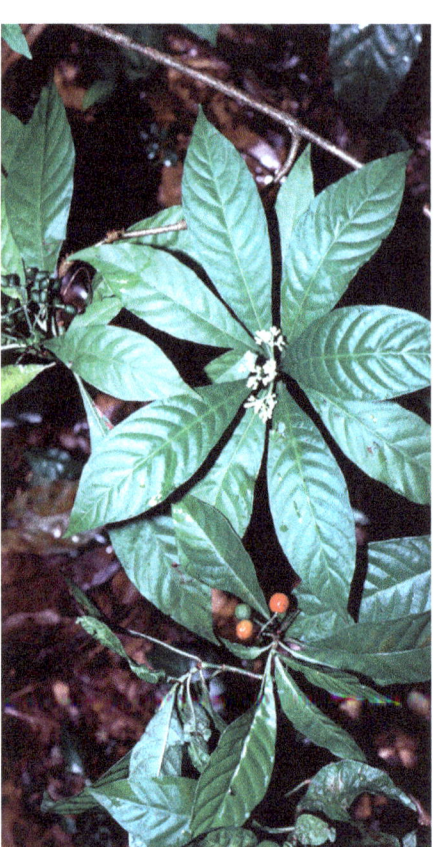

St. John's bush

Spermacoce verticillata L.
Buttonweed
Family: Rubiaceae
Local Preparation: A hot infusion of the leaves for colds.
Bioactive Chemical Profile: Alkaloids (ementine, borrerine and borreverine), terpenes, iridoids, phenolics and flavonoids. (192)
Pharmacological Activity: Ementine has been reported to inhibit Human immunodeficiency virus (HIV) replication. (119)

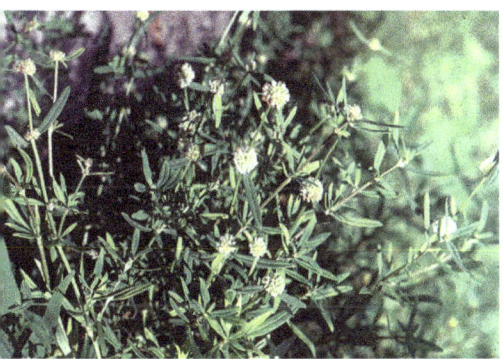

Buttonweed

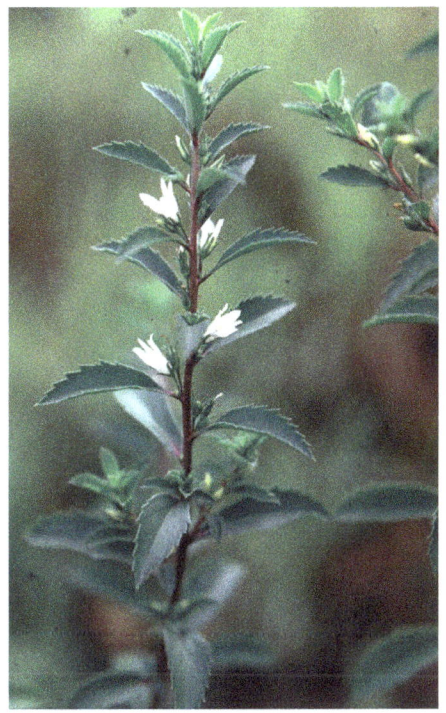

West Indian tea

Capraria biflora L.
West Indian Tea (1)
Family: Scrophulariaceae
Local Preparation: Used in a tonic or cold infusion preparation for colds.
Bioactive Chemical Profile: Two chlorinated iridoids (3-hydroxymyopochlorin and 5-hydroxyglutinoside), five known iridoid glycosides, two flavonoid glucuronides and the phenylethanoid glycoside verbascoside were found in aerial parts of the plant. An o-naphthoquinone, biflorin has also been isolated. (122)(123)
Pharmacological Activity: Biflorin has shown to be a moderate inhibitor of Dengue virus (DENV) protease with an apparent IC_{50} of 89.6 ± 4.4 µM. (193)

Scoparia dulcis L.
Sweet Broom; Licorice Weed
Family: Scrophulariaceae
Local Preparation: Hot infusion or decoction of various parts of the plant.
Bioactive Chemical Profile: Coumarins, phenols, saponins, tannins, amino acids, flavonoids, terpenoids, diterpenoids (e.g. scopadulcic acid) and catecholamines. (70)

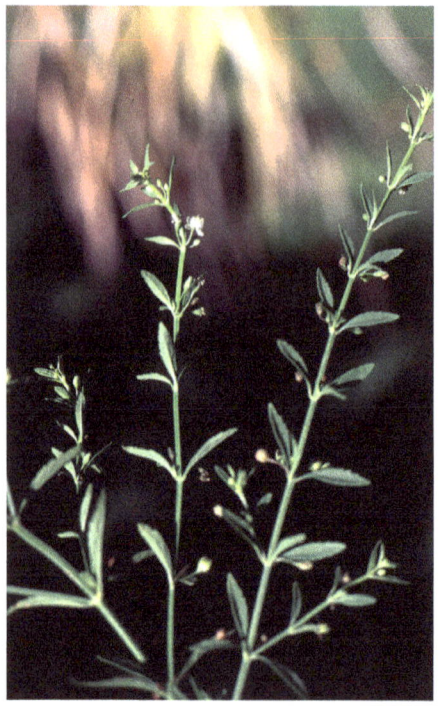

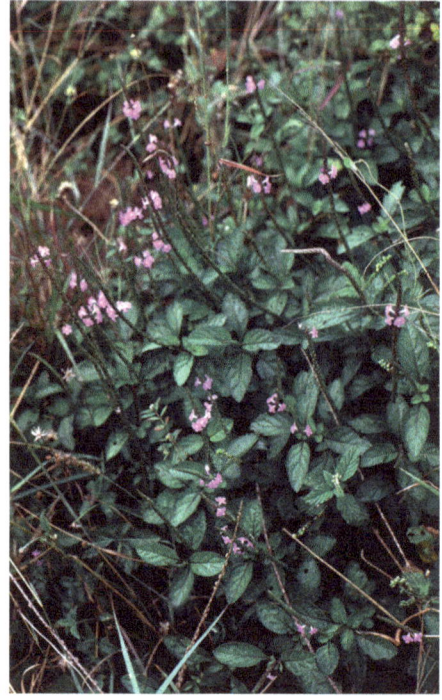

Sweet Broom; Licorice Weed

Vervain

Pharmacological Activity: *In vitro* and *in vivo* antiviral activities of scopadulcic acid B, a diterpenoid from *Scoparia dulcis*, against Herpes simplex virus type-1 with an *in vitro* therapeutic index of 16.7 have been reported. (194)

Pharmacological Activity: An inhibitory action of *S. jamaicensis* against Human immunodeficiency virus-1 (HIV-1) reverse transcriptase along with a strong anti-pyretic effect with efficacy similar to paracetamol have been reported. (196, 197)

Stachytarpheta jamaicensis (L.) Vahl [DC003]
Vervain
Family: Scrophulariaceae
Local Preparation: A hot infusion of the leaves for influenza.
Bioactive Chemical Profile: Alkaloids, coumarins, flavonoids, phenols, saponins, steroids, tannins and terpenoids. (195)

Lantana camara L. [DC019]
Sage
Family: Verbenaceae
Local Preparation: A hot infusion of the young leaves for influenza.
Bioactive Chemical Profile: Essential oils, phenolic compounds, proteins, alkaloids, and carbohydrates (glycosides, oligosaccharides and iridoid glycosides) phenylethanoid,

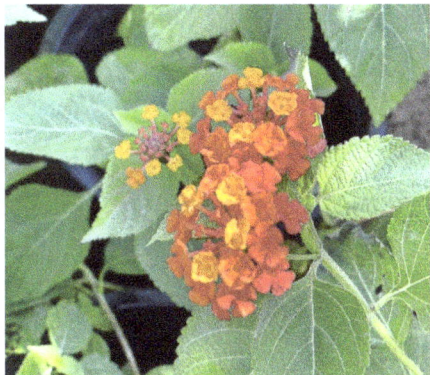

Sage

quinine, saponins, steroids, triterpenes, sesquiterpenoids and tannins. (198)
Pharmacological Activity: The plant's hexane extract at a concentration range of 0.05 and 0.1 mg/ml exhibited the restriction of replication of the Influenza A/Puerto Rico/8/34 (PR8) virus. (199)

Priva lappulacea (L.) Pers.
Velvet Burr
Family: Verbenaceae
Local Preparation: Hot infusion which can be administered with other herbs.
Bioactive Chemical Profile: Ursolic acid, β-sitosterol, luteolin and phenylpropanoids. (200)
Pharmacological Activity: A plant extract with the identified phytochemical(s) exhibited antiviral activity against dengue virus and suppressed replication of influenza A virus. Luteolin inhibits the replication of all four serotypes of dengue virus, but the selectivity of

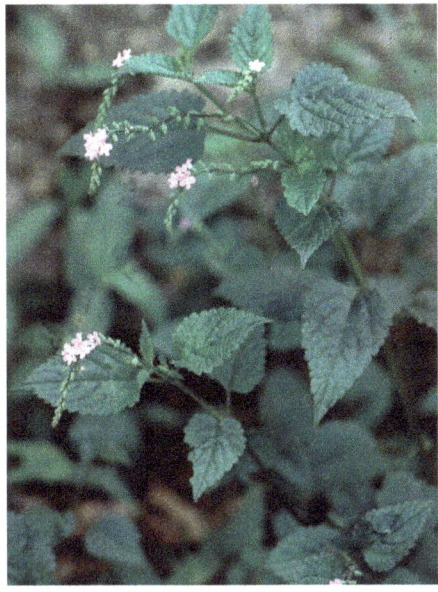

Velvet Burr

the inhibition was weak. Luteolin was also found to reduce infectious virus particle formation, but not viral RNA synthesis, in a hepatoyte derived cellular carcinoma cell line (Huh-7). (201, 202)

FUNGAL INFECTIONS

Asclepias curassavica L
Indian Root, Red Head
Family: Apocynaceae
Local Preparation: Extract of the leaf or crushed leaves (poultice) for topical treatment of ringworm.
Bioactive Chemical Profile: Flavonols, flavonol glycosides, triterpenes, cardenolides, polyphenols, flavonoids, phenols, quinines, tannin, terpenoid, sugars, xanthoprotein, saponin and steroids. (203)

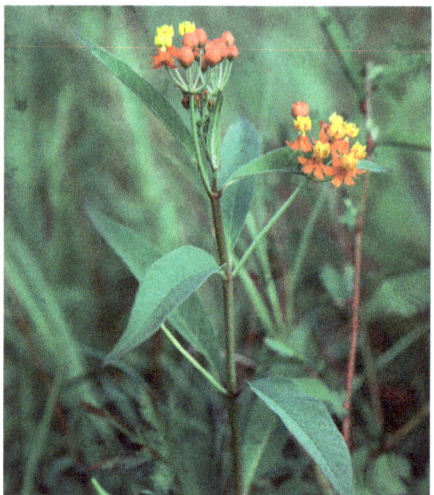

Indian Root, Red Head

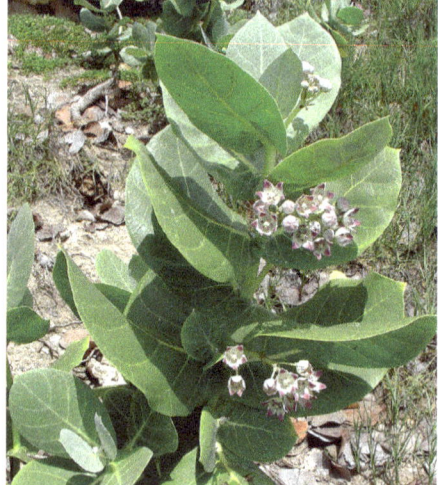

French cotton

Pharmacological Activity: The chloroform extract of the roots of *A. curassavica* derived from Soxhlet extraction, and the water extracts from Soxhlet and cold percolation demonstrated antifungal effects against *Candida albicans*. The latex sap has terpens, cardenolids and glucanases which have been reported to exert antifungal activity. (203, 204)

Calotropis procera (Aiton) iton f.
French Cotton (1)
Family: Apocynaceae
Local Preparation: Latex of the plant applied to the skin for the treatment of ringworm.
Bioactive Chemical Profile: Calotropin, calotropagenin, calotoxin, calactin, uscharin, amyrin, amyrin esters, uscharidin, coroglaucigenin, frugoside, corotoxigenin, calotropagenin, voruscharine and cysteines peptidases. (16, 205)

Pharmacological Activity: Cysteine peptidases extracted from the plant promoted membrane permeabilisation, morphological changes with leakage of cellular content and induction of reactive oxygen species (ROS) in *Fusarium oxysporum* spores. All peptidases were deleterious to the two fungi tested, with IC_{50} of approximately 50 μg/mL. (205)

Jatropha curcas L.
Physic Nut, Monkey Fat Pork (1)
Family: Euphorbiacae
Local Preparation: A preparation of the oils from the seeds.
Bioactive Chemical Profile: Phenols, tannins, phorbol esters, free amino acids and phytic acid were found in various parts of the plant. Seeds contain oils, triacylglycerols, diacylglycerols, monoacylglycerols, free fatty acids, sterols and polar lipids. (110, 206, 207)

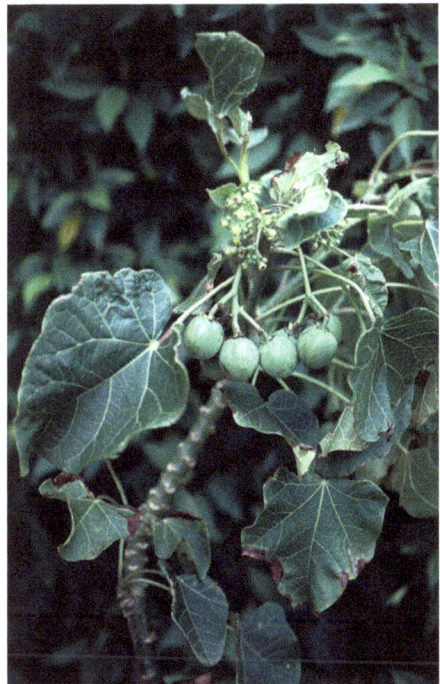
Physic Nut, Monkey Fat Pork

Pharmacological Activity: The phorbol esters in the ethanolic extract of *J. curcas* seed cake demonstrated antifungal activities against important phytofungal pathogens inclusive of *Fusarium oxysporum, Pythium aphanidermatum, Lasiodiplodia theobromae, Curvularia lunata, Fusarium semitectum* with a potency (EC_{50}) of 580 mg/l. Antifungal effects were also reported against *Colletotrichum capsici* and *Colletotrichum gloeosporiodes*. Complete inhibition of the growth of *F. semitectum* and *P. aphanidermatum* was at a concentration of 3000mg/l. (207)

Chamaesyce hirta (L.) Millisp [DC016]
Milk Weed (1)
Family: Euphorbiacae
Local Preparation: Latex of the plant used for the treatment of ringworm.
Bioactive Chemical Profile:
Triterpene and taraxerol have been isolated from the stems. Phytol and phytyl fatty acid esters have been yielded from the leaves; the roots contain cycloartenyl fatty acid ester, lupeol fatty acid ester, α-amyrin fatty acid ester and β-amyrin fatty acid ester, linoleic acid, β-sitosterol and squalene. (112)
Pharmacological Activity: The methanolic leaf extract of *C. hirta* demonstrated antifungal effects against *Candida albicans* with a minimum inhibitory concentration of 3.12 mg/ml via the agar disc diffusion method. (208)

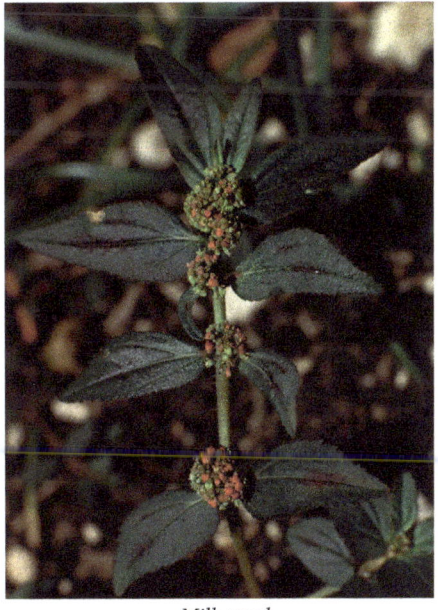
Milk weed

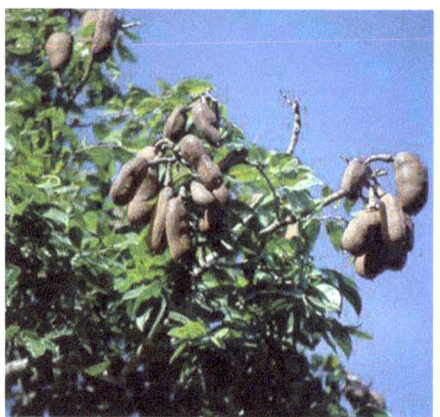
Locust Tree, Stinking Toe Tree

Hymenaea courbaril L.
Locust Tree, Stinking Toe Tree (1)
Family: Fabaceae
Local Preparation: Extract of the leaf and bark for topical treatment of skin ailments.
Bioactive Chemical Profile: Saponins, flavonoids (fisetin & astilbin), coumarins and terpenes. (173, 174, 209)
Pharmacological Activity: The xylem sap of *H. courbaril* inhibited the growth of dermatophytes and of *Candida neoformans* with minimal inhibition concentration (MIC) of <256 ug/ml, while the fisetin, a naturally extracted compound from *H. courbaril*, showed a MIC <128 ug/ml. (209)

Senna alata (L.) Roxb.
Christmas Candle (1)
Family: Fabaceae
Local Preparation: Extract of the leaf or crushed leaves for topical treatment of ringworm.

Bioactive Chemical Profile: Tannins, alkaloids, flavonoids, terpenes, anthraquinone, saponins, phenolics, cannabinoid alkaloids, 1,8-cineole, caryophyllene, limonene, α-selinene, β-caryophyllene, germacrene D, cinnamic acid, pyrazol-5-ol, methaqualone, isoquinoline, quinones, reducing sugars, steroids and volatile oils. (210, 211)

Pharmacological Activity: Several bioactive compounds isolated from the flowers, leaves and bark of *S. alata* exhibit strong *in vitro* and *in vivo* antifungal activities. Extracts tested at a concentration of 500 ug/ml produced antimicrobial activities in *in vitro* assays against *Candida albicans*. (210, 211)

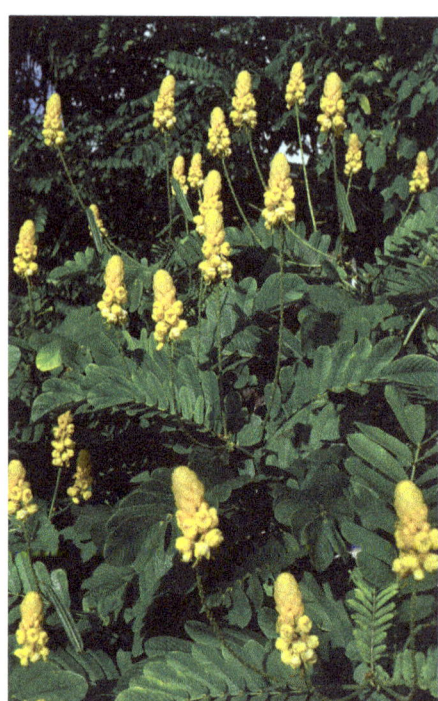
Christmas Candle

BARBADIAN MEDICINAL PLANTS USED BY LOCALS FOR CONDITIONS OTHER THAN COMMUNICABLE AND NON-COMMUNICABLE DISEASES

GIT AILMENTS

Annona muricata L.
Soursop
Family: Annonaceae
Local Preparation: Hot infusion of the leaves to alleviate constipation. (1)
Bioactive Chemical Profile: Tannins and soluble dietary fibres. (212, 213)

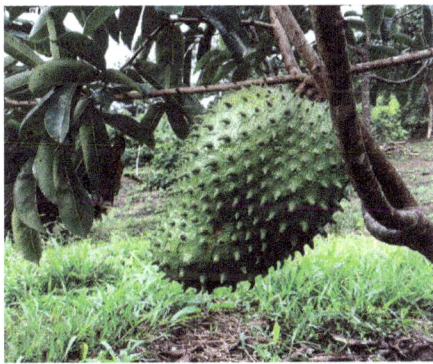

Soursop

Pharmacological Activity: The hydroalcoholic extract of the leaves of *A. muricata* administered at a dose range of 200–400 mg/kg orally showed significant gastroprotective effects in animal ulcerogenic models mediated by endogenous gastric prostaglandin. Rich dietary fiber and tannin content can increase gastrointestinal motility and induce faster gastric emptying. (212–214)

Aloe vera (L.) Burm.f. [DC009]
Aloe
Family: Asphodelaceae
Local Preparation: Eaten raw to purge. (1) The root used as a stomach tonic. (2)
Bioactive Chemical Profile: Aloin and acemannan. (215, 216)
Pharmacological Activity: Studies have confirmed that the ethanolic leaf extract of Aloe vera (50, 100, and 200 mg/kg body weight/day) improved intestinal motility, increased fecal volume, and normalized body weight in constipated rats. The extract of the leaves also reduces abdominal pain/discomfort and improves gastrointestinal health. (215–217)

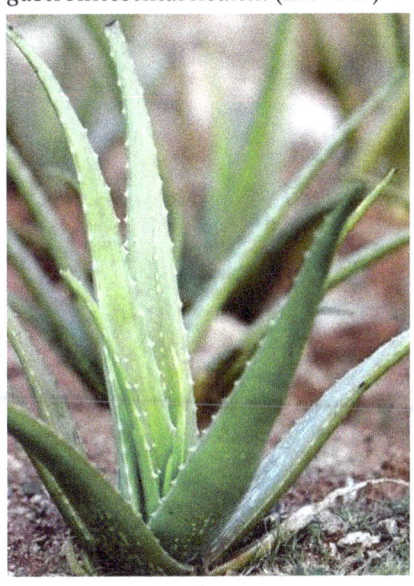

Aloe vera

MEDICINAL PLANTS OF BARBADOS

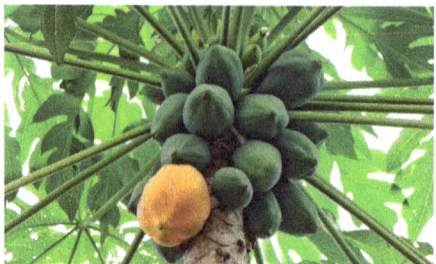
Pawpaw, Papaya

Carica papaya L.[DC011]
Pawpaw, Papaya
Family: Caricaceae
Local Preparation: Fruit eaten ripe to alleviate constipation. (1)
Bioactive Chemical Profile: Soluble dietary fibre and tannins. (218)
Pharmacological Activity: Dietary fibre reduces constipation.

Azadirachta indica A. Juss.
Neem
Family: Meliaceae
Local Preparation: Infusion of the leaves used as a purgative. (2)

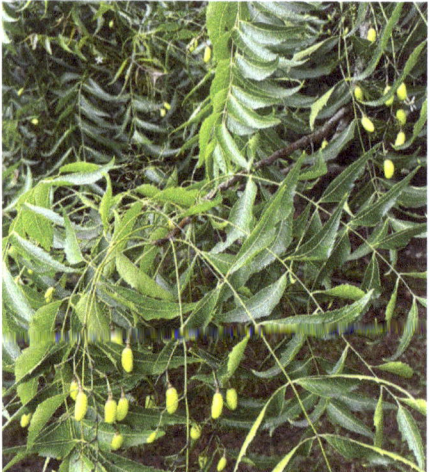
Neem

Bioactive Chemical Profile: Quercetin, kaempferol, myricetin and luteolin. (219)
Pharmacological Activity: A polar extract of *A. indica* and quercetin inhibited the contraction of the isolated rat ileum (small intestine) induced by potassium chloride (KCL) up to 29% and 18%, respectively, and decreased calcium chloride ($CaCl_2$)-induced contraction in the same tissue. This effect supports the use of the plant as a regulator of gastric motility. (219)

Myristica fragrans Houtt.
Nutmeg
Family: Myristicaceae
Local Preparation: Seeds grated and steeped for upset stomach. (1)
Bioactive Chemical Profile: Eugenol and macelignan. (220, 221)
Pharmacological Activity: Eugenol inhibited the growth of 30 *Helicobacter pylori* strains at a concentration of 2 μg/ml after the 9th hour of incubation and may provide gastroprotective

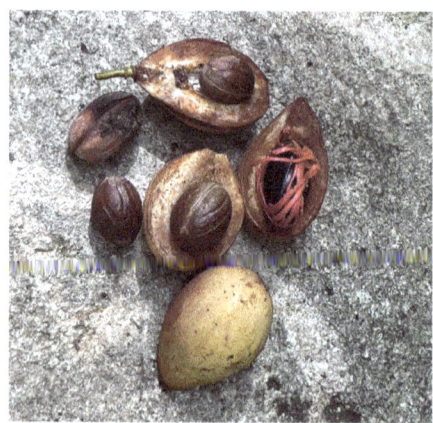
Nutmeg

effects against ulceration. Also, nutmeg is a potent inhibitor of prostaglandin synthesis and a non-selective depressant of the gastric muscles to prostaglandins. (222, 223)

Pimenta racemosa (Mill.) J.W. Moore [DC018]
Bay Leaf
Family: Myrtaceae
Local Preparation: Hot infusion of the leaves taken for upset stomach. (1)
Bioactive Chemical Profile: Terpenoids, steroids, saponins, phenolic nuclei, glycosides, tannins and quinines. (62)
Pharmacological Activity: The aqueous methanol extract of *P. racemosa* leaves at 125, 250 and 500 mg/kg reduced the gastric mucosal lesions compared with the negative control and ranitidine-treated group of animals. The extract also demonstrated increased hepatoprotective effects by reducing circulating levels of alanine aminotransferase (ALT) at three doses and aspartate aminotransferase (AST) only at 125 and 250 mg/kg when compared with the Paracetamol group in lab animals. (63)

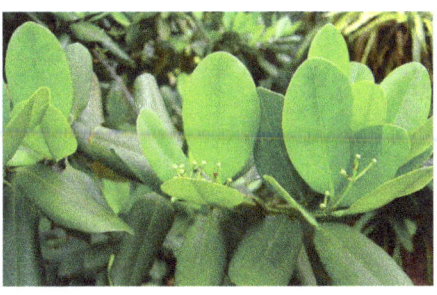

Bay Leaf

Cymbopogon citratus (DC.) Stapf [DC001]
Lemongrass
Family: Poaceae
Local Preparation: Hot infusion of the leaves for diverticulitis. (1)
Bioactive Chemical Profile: Luteolin glycosides and citral. (224, 225)

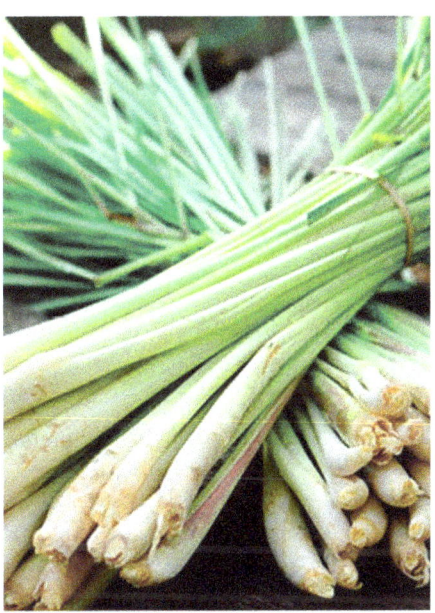

Lemongrass

Pharmacological Activity: Citral at doses between 0.061 mM to 15.6 mM and an extract of *C. Citratus* leaves at doses between 0.001 mg/ml to 1 mg/ml significantly reduced the spontaneous, acetylcholine (ACh) and potassium chloride (KCl) induced ileal contractions in rabbits. Both citral and leaf extract demonstrate spasmolytic activity. (224, 225)

MEDICINAL PLANTS OF BARBADOS

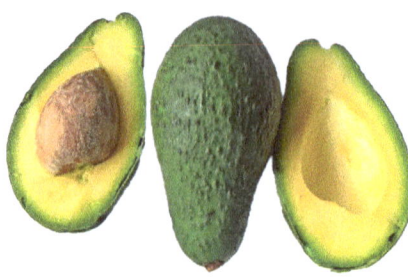

Pear

Persea americana Mill.
Pear
Family: Lauraceae
Local Preparation: A hot infusion of the leaves to alleviate diarrhea. (1) The leaves are also boiled for purgative effects. (1)
Bioactive Chemical Profile: Alkanols, terpenoid glycosides, various furan ring-containing derivatives, flavonoids and a coumarin. (249)
Pharmacological Activity: The chloroform-methanol extract of the leaves of *P. americana* possesses significant anti-diarrhoeal effect at an oral dose of 200 mg/kg biweekly in rats. This effect was comparable to the standard anti-diarrhoeal drug, hyoscine butylbromide. (226)

Capsicum annum L.
Cayenne pepper
Family: Solanaceae
Local Preparation: An extract of the pepper is used for diverticulitis. (1)
Bioactive Chemical Profile: Capsaicinoids, carotenoids and vitamin E/C. (227)
Pharmacological Activity: Potent anti-inflammatory effects of *C. annum* at a dose of four 150 mg pills/day in patients with irritable bowel syndrome have been demonstrated in a randomized controlled trial. This may explain its use for diverticulitis to alleviate abdominal pain and bloating. (227, 228)

Curcuma longa L.
Turmeric
Family: Zingiberaceae
Local Preparation: A hot infusion of the rhizome is used for upset stomach. (2)
Bioactive Chemical Profile: Curcumin and sodium curcuminate. (229)

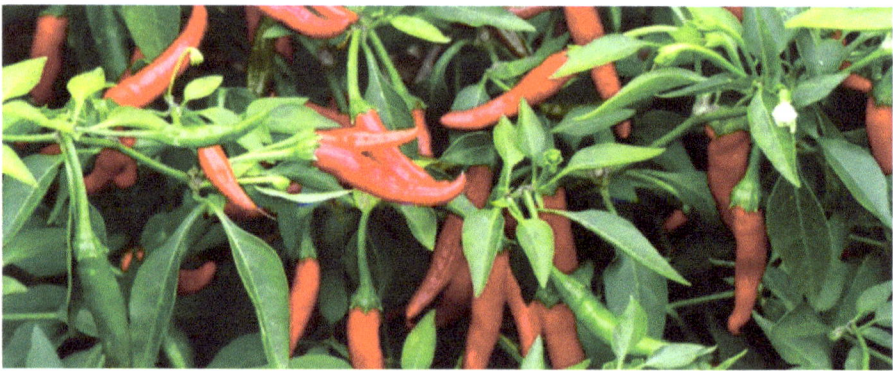

Cayenne pepper

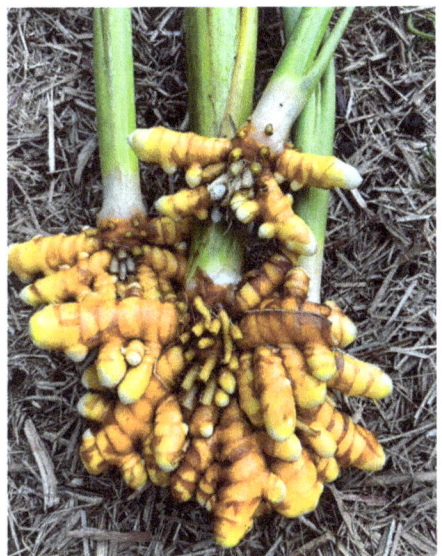

Turmeric

Zingiber officinale Roscoe
Ginger
Family: Zingiberaceae
Local Preparation: Rhizome is grated and steeped or boiled for upset stomach (1) and diverticulitis. (1)
Bioactive Chemical Profile: Gingerol, shogaol, sesquiterpenes and monoterpenes. (230)

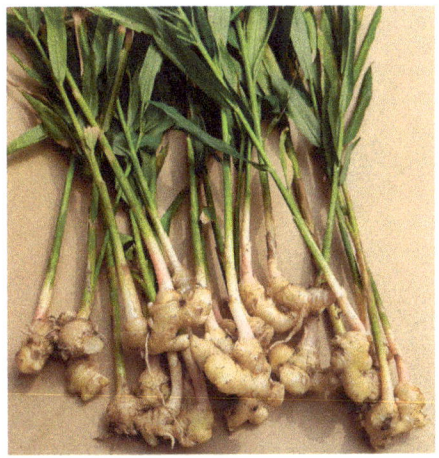

Ginger

Pharmacological Activity: Turmeric is hepatoprotective mainly due to its antioxidant properties, as well as its ability to decrease the formation of proinflammatory cytokines. Sodium curcuminate stimulates bile secretion and thus aids digestion and eliminates toxins from the liver. *C. longa* has also been shown to reduce abdominal pain. In a phase II clinical trial involving 45 subjects with endoscopically diagnosed peptic ulcers, patients were given 600 mg curcumin five times daily for 12 weeks. Ulcers were absent in 12 patients (48%) after four weeks, in 18 patients after eight weeks, and in 19 patients (76%) after 12 weeks. (229)

Pharmacological Activity: Ginger is seen as effective in reducing nausea, vomiting, flatulence, inflammation and increasing gastric emptying. Ginger may reduce nausea and vomiting based on a weak inhibitory effect of gingerols and shogaols at muscarinic (M3) and serotonin 5-HT (3) receptors. Serotonin 5-HT (4) receptors also play a role in gastroduodenal motility. (230, 231).

MEDICINAL PLANTS OF BARBADOS

OTHER CONDITIONS

Justicia secunda Vahl
Bloodroot
Family: Acanthaceae
Local Preparation: A hot infusion is used for cleansing. (2)
Bioactive Chemical Profile: Flavonoids and phenols. (42)

Bllodroot

Pharmacological Activity: A hot extract of *J. secunda* leaves (JSHAE) at a dose range of 100 and 200 mg/kg significantly reduced plasma aspartate aminotransferase, alanine aminotransferase, lactate dehydrogenase and total bilirubin levels following carbon tetrachloride (CCl_4) induced hepatotoxicity compared to untreated rats. JSHAE exhibited significant antioxidant activity. (232)

Allium sativum L.
Garlic
Family: Amaryllidaceae
Local Preparation: A decoction of the leaves is used for muscle/joint pain and circulatory issues.
Bioactive Chemical Profile: Allicin, diallyl sulfide and alliin. (81)
Pharmacological Activity: Garlic supplementation (1000 mg for 8 weeks) significantly improves inflammatory mediators and clinical symptoms, and can be considered as a potential adjunct treatment in rheumatoid arthritis. Other herbal preparations with *A. sativum* improves functional mobility and reduces pain among patients with pain. (233, 234)

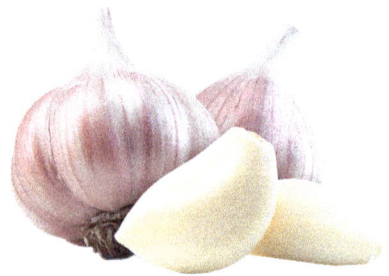

Garlic

Annona muricata L.
Soursop
Family: Annonaceae
Local Preparation: A decoction or hot infusion of the leaves or soaked in water for cooling. A decoction or hot infusion of the leaves for general maintenance of health. (2)
Bioactive Chemical Profile: Acetogenins, phenolic compounds (e.g., cinnamic acid derivatives,

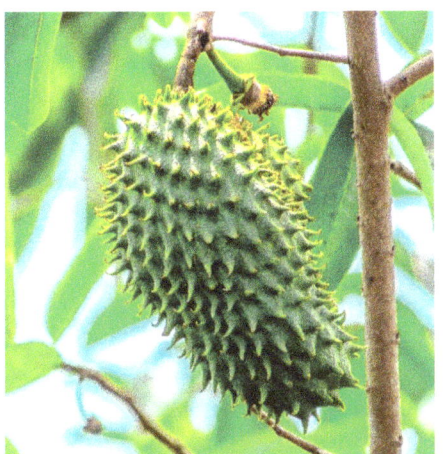
Soursop

p-coumaric acid), reticuline and tannins. (4, 44, 212, 213)
Pharmacological Activity: Various beneficial effects of the leaves and the fruit of soursop have been reported prior; inclusive of antiulcerogenic, anticancer, antihypertensive and laxative effects. (4, 44, 212, 213)

Foeniculum vulgare Mill.
Fennel
Family: Apiaceae
Local Preparation: A hot infusion is used for fever. (2)

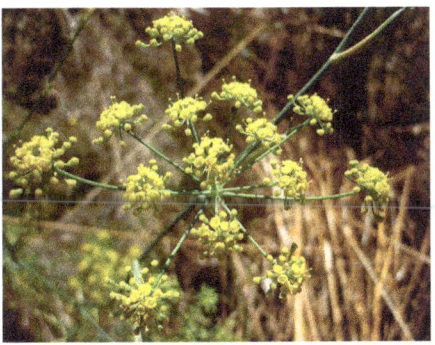
Fennel

Bioactive Chemical Profile: Essential oils inclusive of α-thujene, 1,8-cineol, β-ocimene and linalool, phenolic compounds, fatty acids and amino acids. (235)
Pharmacological Activity: Herbal formulation containing *F. vulgare* showed significant reduction in yeast-induced elevated temperature at a dose of 240mg/kg as compared with that of the standard drug paracetamol. (236)

Petroselinum crispum (Mill.) Fuss
Parsley
Family: Apiaceae
Local Preparation: A decoction of the leaves for general maintenance of health. (2)

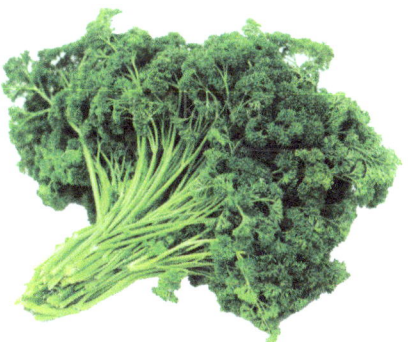
Parsley

Bioactive Chemical Profile: Parsley contains volatile compounds such as terpenes and terpenoids in its essential oil, as well as phenolic compounds in the crude plant extract. (257)
Pharmacological Activity: Parsley's essential oil (0.01–100 μg/ml) suppressed the cellular and humoral immune response. It can also suppress

both nitric oxide (NO) production and the functions of macrophages as the main innate immune cells. (237)

Cocos nucifera L.
Coconut
Family: Arecaceae
Local Preparation: Coconut water is mixed with Epsom salt for cooling. (2)
Bioactive Chemical Profile: The coconut fiber's ethanolic extract has the presence of phenols, tannins, leucoanthocyanidins, flavonoids, triterpenes, steroids, and alkaloids, while a butanol extract recovered triterpenes, saponins and condensed tannins. (258)
Pharmacological Activity: Coconut is known to have wide range of wellness and medicinal benefits. These include analgesic, antiarthritic, antibacterial, antipyretic, antihelminthic, antidiarrheal, and hypoglycemic activities. (258)

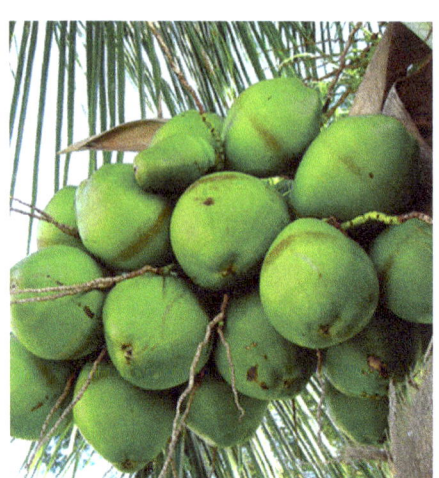

Coconut

Aloe vera (L.) Burm.f. [DC009]
Aloes
Family: Asphodelaceae
Local Preparation: A hot infusion or decoction of the leaves or the sap eaten raw or consumed as a juice for general maintenance of health. A decoction of the leaves or eaten raw for cleansing. (2)
Bioactive Chemical Profile: Acemannan, lupeol and saponin glycosides. (130)
Pharmacological Activity: Emollient, purgative, anti-microbial, anti-inflammatory, antioxidant, aphrodisiac, anti-helmenthic, antifungal, antiseptic and cosmetic effects of *A. vera*'s phytoconstituents have been reported. (130)

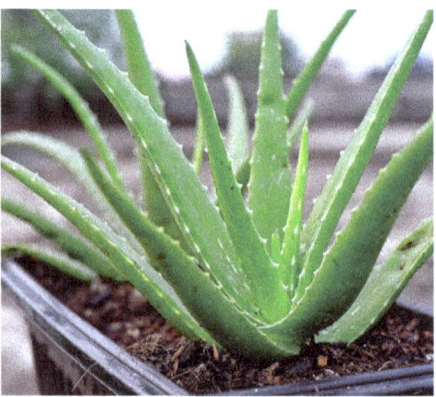

Aloes

Momordica charantia L. [DC002]
Cerasee
Family: Cucurbitaceae
Local Preparation: A decoction of the leaves and stems with sugar for general maintenance of health and for cleansing. (2)

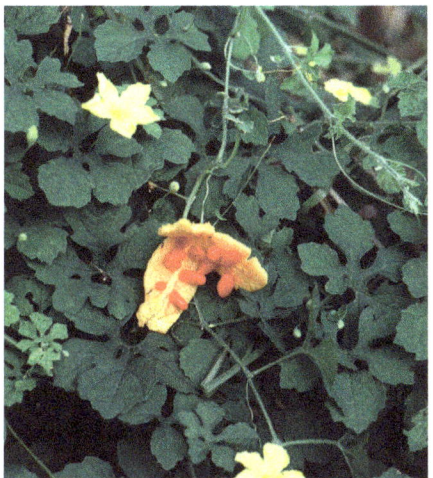
Cerasee

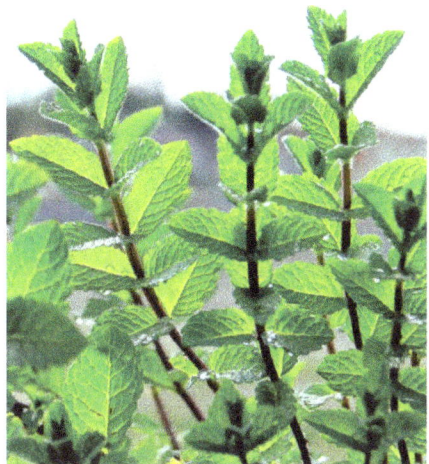
Peppermint

Bioactive Chemical Profile: Triterpenoids and polysaccharides. (238)
Pharmacological Activity: The plant has common pharmacological activities including antimicrobial, antimutagenic, antifertility, antidiabetic, antioxidant, antilipolytic, hypoglycemic, anticancer, antimicrobial, antiviral and hepatoprotective activities. (238)

Mentha x piperita L.
Peppermint
Family: Lamiaceae
Local Preparation: A hot infusion of the leaves for cooling. (2)
Bioactive Chemical Profile: Menthol. (239)
Pharmacological Activity: Antipyretic effects of menthol and peppermint have been demonstrated in a variety of conditions. The menthol receptor, TRPM8, is the predominant thermoceptor for cellular and behavioral responses to cold temperatures. TRPM8 has an emerging role in a variety of biological systems, including thermoregulation, cancer, bladder function and asthma. (239)

Persea americana Mill.
Pear
Family: Lauraceae
Local Preparation: A hot infusion or decoction of the leaves is used for cooling. (2)
Bioactive Chemical Profile: Alkanols, terpenoid glycosides, various furan ring-containing derivatives, flavonoids and a coumarin. (249)

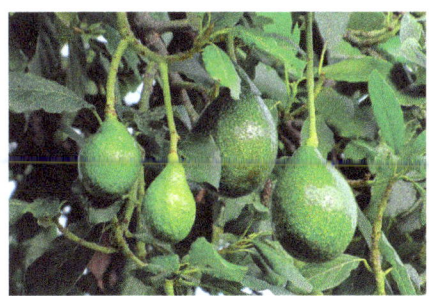
Pear

Pharmacological Activity: The pear plant's extracts have been tested preclinically *in vitro* and *in vivo* and have validated their analgesic and anti-inflammatory activity, hypotensive activity, anticonvulsant effect, antihepatotoxic activity, antioxidant activity and hypoglycaemic effects. (249)

Azadirachta indica A. Juss.
Neem bush
Family: Meliaceae
Local Preparation: A hot infusion of the leaves is used for cleansing. A decoction of the leaves is used for muscle/joint pain. (2)
Bioactive Chemical Profile: Azadiradione, azadirachtin, quercetin and nimbin. (240, 241)
Pharmacological Activity: The carbon tetrachloride extract (CTCE) of *Azadirachta indica* fruit skin and azadiradione, a phytoconstituent, at 100 mg/kg exhibited significant anti-nociceptive and anti-inflammatory activities in animal models. Also, antimicrobial, antiparasitic and antioxidant effects of the phytochemicals extracted from *A. indica* have also been noted. (240, 241)

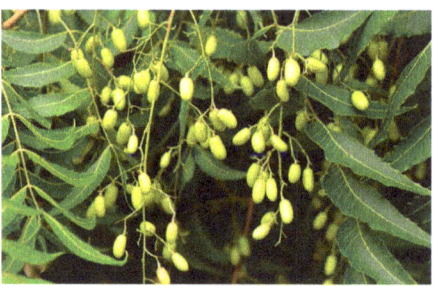

Neem bush

Moringa oleifera Lam.
Moringa
Family: Moringaceae
Local Preparation: A hot infusion or decoction of the leaves or raw nuts consumed for general maintenance of health. A hot infusion or decoction of the leaves is used for cleansing. (2)
Bioactive Chemical Profile: Polysaccharide MOP-2, lauric acid, malic acid and oleic acid. (242)
Pharmacological Activity: Phytochemicals found in *M. oleifera* plant have been shown to regulate the immune system which helps other conditions including cancer, diabetes, and hypertension. *M. oleifera* contributes to the host's health through restructuring the gut microbiota, which in turn helps to control inflammation and enhances host immunity. (242).

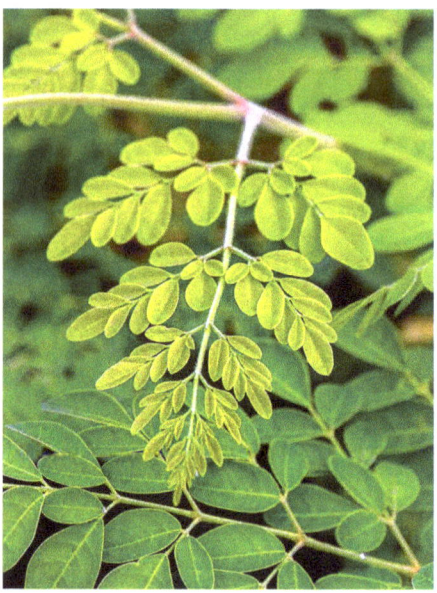

Moringa

Pimenta racemose (Mill.) J.W. Moore L.
Bay Leaf
Family: Myrtaceae
Local Preparation: A hot infusion or decoction of the leaves is used for general maintenance of health. A hot infusion or decoction of the leaves with sugar is consumed for cooling. (2)
Bioactive Chemical Profile: Terpenoids, steroids, saponins, phenolic compounds, glycosides, tannins and quinines. (62)
Pharmacological Activity: Anti-inflammatory, anti-oxidant, anti-pyretic, gastro and hepato-protective and central nervous system depressant effects have been reported prior. (62, 63)

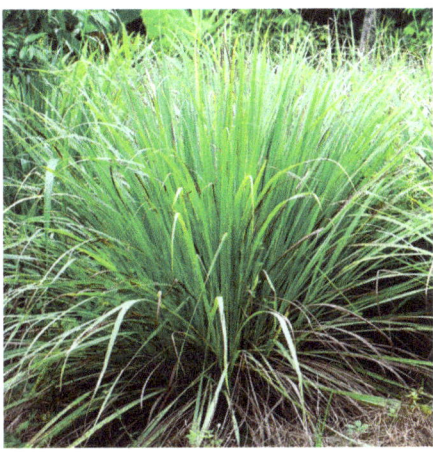

Lemongrass

A decoction of the leaves is used for cooling/fever. (2)
Bioactive Chemical Profile: Essential oils (citral, geranial, neral, β-myrcene, geranyl acetate and isopulegol). (243)
Pharmacological Activity: Remarkable anxiolytic effect of extracts of *C. citratus have been reported* in an animal model. This effect may be related to the modulation of the activity of the $GABA_A$ receptors. Oral administration of the essential oils of *C. citratus* showed dose-dependent anti-inflammatory activity in a carrageenan-induced mouse paw edema model. The anti-inflammatory activity observed at the oral dose of 10 to 100 mg/kg was comparable to the effect using the reference drug diclofenac acid. The antimicrobial efficacy of *C. citratus* against *Salmonella typhi, Salmonella paratyphi* and *Salmonella typhimurium* may support its use to treat enteric fever. (243–245).

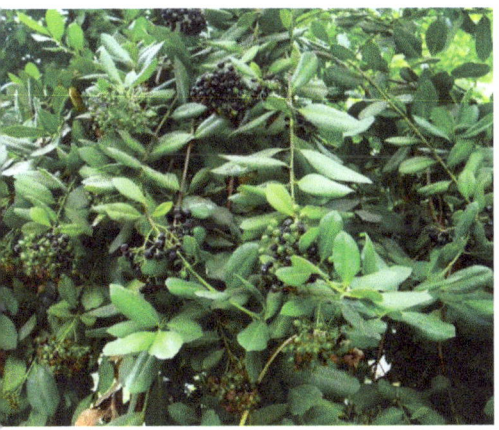

Bay Leaf

Cymbopogon citratus (DC.) Stapf [DC001]
Lemongrass
Family: Poaceae
Local Preparation: A hot infusion or decoction of the leaves is used for general maintenance of health.

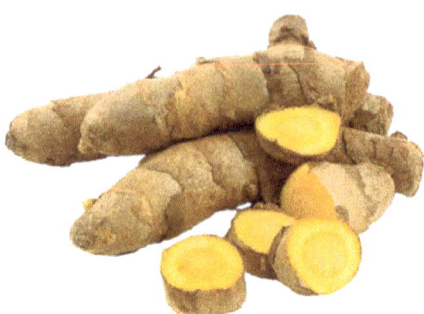

Turmeric

Curcuma longa L.
Ginger
Turmeric
Family: Zingiberaceae
Local Preparation: A hot infusion or decoction of the grated rhizome or tablets/capsule consumed for maintenance of health. A hot infusion or decoction of the leaves is used for muscle/joint pain. A decoction of the rhizome is used for circulation issues. (2)
Bioactive Chemical Profile: Bisdesmethoxyurum, curcumin and desmethoxycurumin. (246)
Pharmacological Activity: *C. longa* was extracted by a systematic solvent method and the extract promoted blood circulation and relieved pain in mice. Curcumins and their derivatives were the major constituents of the extract and were primarily responsible for promotion of blood circulation and relief of pain. (246)

Zingiber officinale Roscoe
Ginger
Family: Zingiberaceae
Local Preparation: A hot infusion or decoction of the grated rhizome is used for general maintenance of health. A hot infusion or decoction of the leaves consumed directly or cooked in a stew for muscle/joint pain. A decoction of the rhizome is used for circulation issues. (2)
Bioactive Chemical Profile: Gingerols and Shagaols. (126)
Pharmacological Activity: *Z. officinale* consumption of 2 grams daily for 11 days largely reduced exercise-induced muscle pain in identical double-blind, placebo controlled, randomized experiments with 34 and 40 volunteers respectively. (247) The ginger crude extract induced vasorelaxation in porcine coronary arteries in an endothelium-dependent manner. The extract also enhanced vasoprotection by the suppression of nitric oxide synthase and cyclooxygenase. (248)

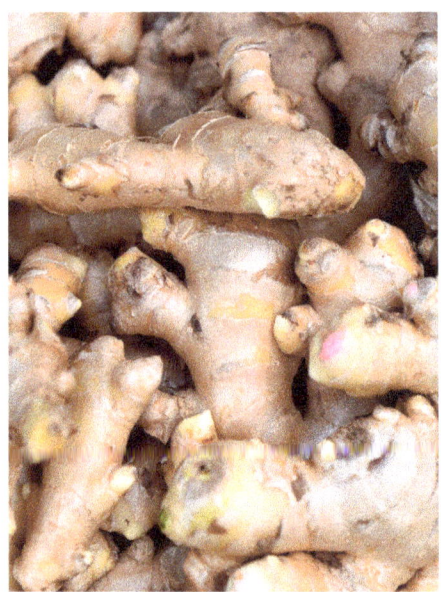

Ginger

Chapter 2 References

1. Sameh S, Al-Sayed E, Labib RM, Singab. AN. Genus Spondias: A phytochemical and pharmacological review. EvidBased Complement Alternat Med. 2018;18.
2. Cohall D. Medicinal Plant Survey Data [Microsoft Excel spreadsheet]. Microsoft Corporation, 2018.
3. Cohall D. Codrington College Lands Project [Video].
4. Yajid AI, Ab Rahman HS, Wong MPK, Wan Zain WZ. Potential benefits of Annona muricata in combating cancer: A review. Malays J Med Sci. 2018;25(1):5–15.
5. Syed Najmuddin SU, Romli MF, Hamid M, Alitheen NB, Nik Abd Rahman NM. Anti-cancer effect of Annona muricata Linn leaves crude extract (AMCE) on breast cancer cell line. BMC Complement Altern Med. 2016;16(1):311.
6. Das S, Sharangi AB. Madagascar perwinkle (Catharantus roseus L.): Diverse medicinal and therapeutic benefits to humankind. J Pharmacogn Phytochem. 2017;6(5):1695–701.
7. Otsuki N, Dang NH, Kumagai E, Kondo A, Iwata S, Morimoto C. Aqueous extract of Carica papaya leaves exhibits anti-tumor activity and immunomodulatory effects. J Ethnopharmacol. 2010;127(3):760–7.
8. Pandey S, Walpole C, Cabot PJ, Shaw PN, Batra J, Hewavitharana AK. Selective anti-proliferative activities of Carica papaya leaf juice extracts against prostate cancer. Biomed Pharmacother. 2017;89:515–23.
9. Patel JR, Tripathi P, Sharma V, Chauhan NS, Dixit VK. Phyllanthus amarus: ethnomedicinal uses, phytochemistry and pharmacology: a review. J Ethnopharmacol. 2011;138(2):286–313.
10. Lee SH, Jaganath IB, Wang SM, Sekaran SD. Antimetastatic effects of Phyllanthus on human lung (A549) and breast (MCF-7) cancer cell lines. PLoS One. 2011;6(6):e20994.

11. Xu S, Li N, Ning MM, Zhou CH, Yang QR, Wang MW. Bioactive compounds from Peperomia pellucida. J Nat Prod. 2006;69(2):247–50.
12. Pappachen L, Chacko A. Preliminary phytochemical screening and in-vitro cytotoxicity activity of Peperomia pellucida Linn. Pharm Glob. 2013;4(8):1–4.
13. Ferreira LM, Vale AEd, Souza AJd, Leite KB, Sacramento C, Moreno ML, et al. Anatomical and phytochemical characterization of Physalis angulata L.: A plant with therapeutic potential. Pharmacogn Res. 2019;11(2):171–7.
14. Hseu YC, Wu CR, Chang HW, Kumar KJ, Lin MK, Chen CS, et al. Inhibitory effects of Physalis angulata on tumor metastasis and angiogenesis. J Ethnopharmacol. 2011;135(3):762–71.
15. Gao CY, Ma T, Luo J, Kong LY. Three new cytotoxic withanolides from the Chinese folk medicine Physalis angulata. Nat Prod Commun. 2015;10(12):2059–62.
16. Balekar N, Parihar G. Calotropis procera: A phytochemical and pharmacological review. Thai J Pharm Sci. 2016;40(3):115–31.
17. Upandhyay R. Ethnomedicinal, pharmaceutical and pesticidal uses of Calotropis procera (Aiton) Family: Asclepiadacae. Int J Green Pharm. 2014;8(8).
18. Sumi FA, Sikder B, Rahman MM, Lubna SR, Ulla A, Hossain MH, et al. Phenolic content analysis of Aloe vera gel and evaluation of the effect of Aloe gel supplementation on oxidative stress and fibrosis in isoprenaline-administered cardiac damage in rats. Prev Nutr Food Sci. 2019;24(3):254–64.
19. Kishore K. Effect of Aloe vera (Aloe barbadensis) on thrombosis in mice. Pharmacologia. 2015;6(8):347–54.
20. Ikeno Y, Hubbard GB, Lee S, Yu BP, Herlihy JT. The influence of long-term Aloe vera ingestion on age-related disease in male Fischer 344 rats. Phytother Res. 2002;16(8):712–8.
21. Zhou Y-X, Xin H-L, Rahman K, Wang S-J, Peng C, Zhang H. Portulaca oleracea L.: A review of phytochemistry and pharmacological effects. Biomed Res Int. 2015;2015.
22. Sabzghabaee AM, Kelishadi R, Jelokhanian H, Asgary S, Ghannadi A, Badri S. Clinical effects of Portulaca Oleracea seeds on Dyslipidemia in obese adolescents: a triple-blinded randomized controlled trial. Med Arch. 2014;68(3):195–9.

23. Chien SC, Young PH, Hsu YJ, Chen CH, Tien YJ, Shiu SY, et al. Anti-diabetic properties of three common Bidens pilosa variants in Taiwan. Phytochemistry. 2009;70(10):1246–54.
24. Ajagun-Ogunleye MO, Tirwomwe M, Mitaki RN, Ejekwumadu JN, Kasozi KI, Pantoglou J, et al. Hypoglycemic and high dosage effects of Bidens pilosa in Type-1 Diabetes Mellitus. J Diabetes Mellit. 2015;5:146–54.
25. Florence NT, Benoit MZ, Jonas K, Alexandra T, Désiré DD, Pierre K, et al. Antidiabetic and antioxidant effects of Annona muricata (Annonaceae), aqueous extract on streptozotocin-induced diabetic rats. J Ethnopharmacol. 2014;151(2):784–90.
26. Bharti SK, Krishnan S, Kumar A, Kumar A. Antidiabetic phytoconstituents and their mode of action on metabolic pathways. Ther Adv Endocrinol Metab. 2018;9(3):81–100.
27. Wang L, Waltenberger B, Pferschy-Wenzig EM, Blunder M, Liu X, Malainer C, et al. Natural product agonists of peroxisome proliferator-activated receptor gamma (PPARγ): a review. Biochem Pharmacol. 2014;92(1):73–89.
28. Li J, Coleman C, Wu H, Burandt C, Ferreira D, Zjawiony J. Triterpenoids and flavonoids from Cecropia schreberiana Miq. (Urticaceae). Biochem Syst Ecol. 2013;48:96–9.
29. Costa GM, Schenkel EP, Reginatto FH. Chemical and pharmacological aspects of the genus Cecropia. Nat Prod Commun. 2011;6(6):913–20.
30. Bortolotti M, Mercatelli D, Polito L. Momordica charantia, a nutraceutical approach for inflammatory related diseases. Front Pharmacol. 2019;10:486.
31. Alam MA, Uddin R, Subhan N, Rahman MM, Jain P, Reza HM. Beneficial role of Bitter Melon supplementation in obesity and related complications in metabolic syndrome. J Lipids. 2015;2015:496169.
32. Bagalkotkar G, Sagineedu SR, Saad MS, Stanslas J. Phytochemicals from Phyllanthus niruri Linn. and their pharmacological properties: a review. J Pharm Pharmacol. 2006;58(12):1559–70.
33. Kaur N, Kaur B, Sirhindi G. Phytochemistry and pharmacology of Phyllanthus niruri L.: A Review. Phytother Res. 2017;31(7):980–1004.
34. Ilango K, Maharajan G, Narasimhan S. Anti-nociceptive and anti-inflammatory activities of Azadirachta indica fruit skin

35. extract and its isolated constituent azadiradione. Nat Prod Res. 2013;27(16):1463–7.
35. Tembe-Fokunang EA, Charles F, Kaba N, Donatien G, Michael A, Bonaventure N. The potential pharmacological and medicinal properties of Neem (Azadirachta indica A. Juss) in the drug development of phytomedicine. J Complement Altern Med Res. 2019;7(1):1–18.
36. Bisht S, Sisodia SS. Anti-hyperglycemic and antidyslipidemic potential of Azadirachta indica leaf extract In STZ- induced diabetes mellitus. J Pharm Sci Res. 2010;2(10):622–7.
37. Shori AB, Baba AS. Antioxidant activity and inhibition of key enzymes linked to type-2 diabetes and hypertension by Azadirachta indica-yogurt. J Saudi Chem Soc. 2013;17(3):295–301.
38. Gupta R, Mathur M, Bajaj VK, Katariya P, Yadav S, Kamal R, et al. Evaluation of antidiabetic and antioxidant activity of Moringa oleifera in experimental diabetes. J Diabetes. 2012;4(2):164–71.
39. Gandhi GR, Vasconcelos ABS, Wu DT, Li HB, Antony PJ, Li H, et al. Citrus flavonoids as promising phytochemicals targeting diabetes and related complications: A systematic review of in vitro and in vivo studies. Nutrients. 2020;12(10).
40. Leal LKAM, Silva AH, Viana GSdB. Justicia pectoralis, a coumarin medicinal plant have potential for the development of antiasthmatic drugs? Revista Brasileira de Farmacognosia. 2017;27(6):794–802.
41. Mpiana PT, Ngbolua KN, Bokota MT, Kasonga TK, Atibu EK, Tshibangu DS, et al. In vitro effects of anthocyanin extracts from Justicia secunda Vahl on the solubility of haemoglobin S and membrane stability of sickle erythrocytes. Blood Transfus. 2010;8(4):248–54.
42. Koffi EN, Guerneve CL, Lozano PR, Meudec E, Adje FA, Bekro YA, et al. Polyphenol extraction and characterization of Justicia secunda Vahl leaves for traditional medicinal uses. Ind Crop Prod. 2013;49:682–9.
43. Manda P, Abrogoua DP, Bahi C, Dano DS, Gnahoui G, Kablan BJ. Evaluation of the antihypertensive activity of total aqueous extract of Justicia secunda Vahl (Acanthaceae). Afr J Pharm Pharmacol 2011;5(16):1838–45.
44. Adefegha SA, Oyeleye SI, Oboh G. Distribution of phenolic contents, antidiabetic potentials, antihypertensive properties, and

antioxidative effects of Soursop (Annona muricata L.) fruit parts in vitro. Biochem Res Int. 2015;2015:347673.
45. Nwokocha CR, Owu DU, Gordon A, Thaxter K, McCalla G, Ozolua RI, et al. Possible mechanisms of action of the hypotensive effect of Annona muricata (soursop) in normotensive Sprague-Dawley rats. Pharm Biol. 2012;50(11):1436–41.
46. Ajebli M, Eddouks M. Antihypertensive activity of Petroselinum crispum through inhibition of vascular calcium channels in rats. J Ethnopharmacol. 2019;242:112039.
47. Dimo T, Rakotonirina SV, Tan PV, Azay J, Dongo E, Cros G. Leaf methanol extract of Bidens pilosa prevents and attenuates the hypertension induced by high-fructose diet in Wistar rats. J Ethnopharmacol. 2002;83(3):183–91.
48. Pino J, Marbot R, Payo A, Chao D, Herrera P, Martí M. Leaf oils of two Cuban Asteraceae species: Pluchea carolinensis Jacq. and Ambrosia hispida Pursh. J Essent Oil Res. 2005;17:318–20.
49. Murugeasn S, Kumar S, Raja B. Antihypertensive and antioxidant potential of Borneol-A natural Terpene in L-NAME – induced hypertensive rats. Int J Pharm Biol Arch. 2010;1:271–9.
50. Santana LF, Inada AC, Espirito Santo B, Filiú WFO, Pott A, Alves FM, et al. Nutraceutical potential of Carica papaya in metabolic syndrome. Nutrients. 2019;11(7).
51. Hasimun P, Sulaeman A, Maharani IDP. Supplementation of Carica papaya leaves (Carica papaya L.) in Nori preparation reduced blood pressure and arterial stiffness on hypertensive animal model. J Young Pharm. 2020;12(1):63–6.
52. Anand V. An updated review of Terminalia catappa. Phcog Rev. 2015;9:93–8.
53. Oyeleye S, Adebayo A, Ogunsuyi O, Dada FA, Oboh G. Phenolic profile and enzyme inhibitory activities of Almond (Terminalia catappa) leaf and stem bark. Int J Food Prop. 2018;20:1–12.
54. Meena J, Sharma RA, Rolania R. A review on Phytochemical and Pharmacological Properties of Phyllanthus amarus Schum. and Thonn. Int J Pharm Sci Res. 2017;9(4):1377–86.
55. Yao NA, Niazi ZR, Najmanová I, Kamagaté M, Said A, Chabert P, et al. Preventive beneficial effect of an aqueous extract of Phyllanthus amarus Schum. and Thonn. (Euphorbiaceae) on DOCA-salt-induced

hypertension, cardiac hypertrophy and dysfunction, and endothelial dysfunction in rats. J Cardiovasc Pharmacol. 2020;75(6):573–83.
56. Bello I, Usman NS, Dewa A, Abubakar K, Aminu N, Asmawi MZ, et al. Blood pressure lowering effect and vascular activity of Phyllanthus niruri extract: The role of NO/cGMP signaling pathway and β-adrenoceptor mediated relaxation of isolated aortic rings. J Ethnopharmacol. 2020;250:112461.
57. Ma X, Zheng C, Hu C, Rahman K, Qin L. The genus Desmodium (Fabaceae)-traditional uses in Chinese medicine, phytochemistry and pharmacology. J Ethnopharmacol. 2011;138:314–32.
58. Parthasarathy R, Singh A, Bhowmik D. A study on preliminary phytochemical and diuretic activity of bark of Thespesia populnea. Int J Pharm Sci Res. 2010;1(2):72–7.
59. Rajbanshi SL, Paranjape A, Sangeetha C, Rajbanshi L. Evaluation of cardioprotective effect of Thespesia populnea with special reference to antioxidant activity [Dissertation]. Ahmedabad, India: Gujarat Technological University; 2018.
60. Chaves OS, Teles YC, Monteiro MM, Mendes Junior LD, Agra MF, Braga VA, et al. Alkaloids and phenolic compounds from Sida rhombifolia L. (Malvaceae) and vasorelaxant activity of two indoquinoline alkaloids. Molecules. 2017;22(1).
61. Aekthammarat D, Pannangpetch P, Tangsucharit P. Moringa oleifera leaf extract lowers high blood pressure by alleviating vascular dysfunction and decreasing oxidative stress in L-NAME hypertensive rats. Phytomedicine. 2019;54:9–16.
62. Contreras B, Rojas J, Lucero M, Celis MT. Preliminary phytochemical screening of Pimenta racemosa var. racemosa (Myrtaceae) from Táchira—Venezuela. Pharmacologyonline. 2014;2:61–8.
63. Moharram FA, Al-Gendy AA, El-Shenawy SM, Ibrahim BM, Zarka MA. Phenolic profile, anti-inflammatory, antinociceptive, anti-ulcerogenic and hepatoprotective activities of Pimenta racemosa leaves. BMC Complement Altern Med. 2018;18(1):208.
64. Ingale AG, Hivrale AU. Pharmacological studies of Passiflora sp. and their bioactive compounds. Afr J of Plant Sc. 2010;4(10):417–26.
65. Ichimura T, Yamanaka A, Ichiba T, Toyokawa T, Kamada Y, Tamamura T, et al. Antihypertensive effect of an extract of Passiflora edulis rind in spontaneously hypertensive rats. Biosci Biotechnol Biochem. 2006;70(3):718–21.

66. Nwokocha CR, Owu DU, Kinlocke K, Murray J, Delgoda R, Thaxter K, et al. Possible mechanism of action of the hypotensive effect of Peperomia pellucida and interactions between human cytochrome P450 enzymes. Med Aromat Plants. 2012;1(4).
67. Mun'Im A, Ramadhani F, Chaerani K, Amelia L, Arrahman A. Effects of gamma irradiation on microbiological, phytochemical content, antioxidant activity and inhibition of angiotensin converting enzyme (ACE) activity of Peromia pellucida (L.) Kunth. J Young Pharm. 2017;9(1s):S65–S9.
68. Najafian Y, Hamedi SS, Farshchi MK, Feyzabadi Z. Plantago major in traditional Persian medicine and modern phytotherapy: a narrative review. Electron Physician. 2018;10(2):6390–9.
69. Nyunt TM, Lwin KK, Aye TT, Than MA, Chit K, Kyaw T, et al. Antihypertensive effect of Plantago major Linn. whole plant (Ahkyawpaung-tahtaung) on mild to moderate hypertensive patients. Myanmar Health Sci Res J. 2007;19:97–102.
70. Murti K, Panchai M, Taya P, Singh R. Pharmacological Properties of Scoparia Dulcis: A Review. Pharmacologia. 2012;3(8):344–7.
71. Sarkar A, Ghosh P, Poddar S, Sarkar T, Choudhury S, Chatterjee S. Phytochemical, botanical and ethnopharmacological study of Scoparia dulcis Linn. (Scrophulariaceae): A concise review. J Pharm Innov. 2020;9(7):30–5.
72. Rengifo-Salgado E, Vargas-Arana G. Physalis angulata L. (Bolsa Mullaca): A review of its traditional uses, chemistry, and pharmacology. Bol Latinoam Caribe Plantas Med Aromat 2013;12(5):431–45.
73. Nanumala SK, Gunda K, Runja C, Chandra MS. Evaluations of diuretic activity of methanolic extract of Physalis angulata L. leaves. Int J Pharm Sci Rev Res. 2012;16(2):40–2.
74. Simaremare ES, Holle E, Gunawan E, Yabansabra YR, Octavia F, Pratiwi RD. Toxicity, antioxidant, analgesic and anti-inflamantory of ethanol extracts of Laportea aestuans (Linn.) Chew. J Chem Pharm Res. 2018;10(5):16–23.
75. Hussain H, Hussain J, Al-Harrasi A, Shinwari ZK. Chemistry of some species genus Lantana. Pak J Bot. 2011;43(SI):51–62.
76. Setzer WN, Schmidt JM, Noletto JA, Vogler B. Leaf oil compositions and bioactivities of Abaco bush medicines. Pharmacologyonline. 2006;3:794–802.

77. Leong X-F. The spice for hypertension: Protective role of Curcuma longa. Biomed Pharmacol J. 2018;11(4):1829–40.
78. Adjibode AG, Tougan UP, Youssao AKI, Mensah GA, Hanzen C, Koutinhouin GB. Synedrella nodiflora (L.) Gaertn: A review on its phytochemical screening and uses in animal husbandry and medicine. Int J Adv Sci Technol Res. 2015;5(3):436–43.
79. Maiyo ZC, Ngure RM, Matasyoh JC, Chepkorir R. Phytochemical constituents and antimicrobial activity of leaf extract of three Amaranthus plant species. Afr J Biochem. 2009;9.
80. Guo L, Wang Y, Bi X, Duo K, Sun Q, Yun X, et al. Antimicrobial activity and mechanism of action of the Amaranthus tricolor crude extract against Staphylococcus aureus and potential application in cooked meat. Foods. 2020;9(3):359.
81. Shang A, Cao SY, Xu XY, Gan RY, Tang GY, Corke H, et al. Bioactive compounds and biological functions of garlic (Allium sativum L.). Foods. 2019;8(7): 246, doi:10.3390/foods8070246.
82. Zardast M, Namakin K, Esmaelian Kaho J, Hashemi SS. Assessment of antibacterial effect of garlic in patients infected with Helicobacter pylori using urease breath test. Avicenna J Phytomed. 2016;6(5):495–501.
83. Locatelli DA, Nazareno MA, Fusari CM, Camargo AB. Cooked garlic and antioxidant activity: Correlation with organosulfur compound composition. Food Chem. 2017;220:219–24.
84. Nadaf NH, Parulekar RS, Patil RS, Gade TK, Momin AA, Waghmare SR, et al. Biofilm inhibition mechanism from extract of Hymenocallis littoralis leaves. J Ethnopharmacol. 2018;222:121–32.
85. Abou-Donia AH, Toaima SM, Hammoda HM, Shawky E, Kinoshita E, Takayama H. Phytochemical and biological investigation of Hymenocallis littoralis SALISB. Chem Biodivers. 2008;5(2):332–40.
86. Santana O, Reinab M, Anaya AL, Hernández F, Izquierdo ME, González-Coloma A. 3-O-Acetyl-narcissidine, a bioactive alkaloid from Hippeastrum puniceum Lam. (Amaryllidaceae). Z Naturforsch C J Biosci. 2008;63(9–10):639–43.
87. Segaran G, Sathiavelu M. Antibacterial activity of an ornamental plant Hippeastrum fosteri. Bangladesh J Pharmacol. 2021;16(2):49–51.
88. Reddy CU, Reddy KS, Reddy JJ. Aloe vera - a wound healer. Asian J Oral Health Allied Sci. 2011;1(1):91–2.

89. Kamboj A, Saluja AK. Ageratum conyzoides L.: A review on its phytochemical and pharmacological profile. Int J Green Pharm. 2008;2.
90. Shagolsem BS, Devi WR, Devi WI, Swapana N, Chingakham B S. Ethnobotany, phytochemistry and pharmacology of Ageratum conyzoides Linn (Asteraceae). Journal of medicinal plant research. 2013;7.
91. Shandukani PD, Tshidino SC, Masoko P, Moganedi KM. Antibacterial activity and in situ efficacy of Bidens pilosa Linn and Dichrostachys cinerea Wight et Arn extracts against common diarrhoea-causing waterborne bacteria. BMC Complement Altern Med. 2018;18(1):171.
92. Block LC, Santos AR, de Souza MM, Scheidt C, Yunes RA, Santos MA, et al. Chemical and pharmacological examination of antinociceptive constituents of Wedelia paludosa. J Ethnopharmacol. 1998;61(1):85–9.
93. Mizokami SS, Arakawa NS, Ambrosio SR, Zarpelon AC, Casagrande R, Cunha TM, et al. Kaurenoic acid from Sphagneticola trilobata inhibits inflammatory pain: Effect on cytokine production and activation of the NO-cyclic GMP-protein kinase G-ATP-sensitive potassium channel signaling pathway. J Nat Prod. 2012;75(5):896–904.
94. Leite AGB, Farias ETN, Oliveira APd, Abreu REFd, Costa MMd, Almeida JRG, et al. Phytochemical screening and antimicrobial activity testing of crude hydroalcoholic extract from leaves of Sphagneticola trilobata (Asteraceae). Cienc Rural. 2019;49(4).
95. Ghori M, Ghaffari M, Hussain S, Manzoor M, Aziz M, Sarwer W. Ethnopharmacological, phytochemical and pharmacognostic potential of genus Heliotropium L. Turk J Pharm Sci. 2016;13:143–68.
96. Rahimifard N, Bagheri E, Asgarpanah J, Yazdi H, Bagheri F. Study of the antibacterial activity of total extract and petroleum ether, chloroform, ethyl acetate and aqueous fractions of aerial parts of Heliotropium bacciferum against Staphylococcus aureus, Bacillus cereus, Pseudomonas aeruginosa, E.coli, Salmonella enteritidis. Biosci Biotechnol Res Asia. 2014;11:239–48.
97. Fayed MAA. Heliotropium; a genus rich in pyrrolizidine alkaloids: A systematic review following its phytochemistry and pharmacology. Phytomed Plus. 2021;1(2):100036.

98. Chen ML, Wu S, Tsai TC, Wang LK, Chou WM, Tsai FM. The caffeic acid in aqueous extract of Tournefortia sarmentosa enhances neutrophil phagocytosis of Escherichia coli. Immunopharmacol Immunotoxicol. 2014;36(6):390–6.
99. Morteza-Semnani K, Saeedi M, Akbarzadeh M. The essential oil composition of Messerschmidia sibirica L. J Essent Oil Res. 2008;20(3):207–8.
100. Zunjar V, Dash RP, Jivrajani M, Trivedi B, Nivsarkar M. Antithrombocytopenic activity of carpaine and alkaloidal extract of Carica papaya Linn. leaves in busulfan induced thrombocytopenic Wistar rats. J Ethnopharmacol. 2016;181:20–5.
101. Ghosh S, Saha M, Bandyopadhyay PK, Jana M. Extraction, isolation and characterization of bioactive compounds from chloroform extract of Carica papaya seed and its in vivo antibacterial potentiality in Channa punctatus against Klebsiella PKBSG14. Microb Pathog. 2017;111:508–18.
102. Phatak RS. GC-MS analysis of bioactive compounds in the methanolic extract of Kalanchoe pinnata fresh leaves. J Chem Pharm Res. 2015;7(3):34–7.
103. Ebere Okwu D, Uchenna Nnamdi F. A novel antimicrobial phenanthrene alkaloid from Bryopyllum pinnatum. J Chem. 2011;8:972359.
104. Pattewar SV, Patil DN, Dahikar SB. Antimicrobial potential of extract from leaves of Kalanchoe pinnata. Int J Pharm Sci Res. 2013;4(12):4577–80.
105. Nayak BS, Marshall JR, Isitor G. Wound healing potential of ethanolic extract of Kalanchoe pinnata Lam. leaf--a preliminary study. Indian J Exp Biol. 2010;48(6):572–6.
106. Agatemor UM-M, Nwodo OFC, Anosike CA. Anti-inflammatory activity of Cucumis sativus L. J Pharm Res Int. 2015;8(2):1–8.
107. Foong FHN, Aqeelah M, Solachuddin Jauhari Arief I. Biological properties of cucumber (Cucumis sativus L) extracts. Malaysian J Anal Sci. 2015;19(6):1218–22.
108. Ferlemi AV, Lamari FN. Berry leaves: An alternative source of bioactive natural products of nutritional and medicinal value. Antioxidants (Basel). 2016;5(2).
109. Sadowska B, Paszkiewicz M, Podsędek A, Redzynia M, Różalska

110. Laxane S, Swarnkar S, Kenganora M, Zanwar SB, Manganahalli M. Jatropha curcas: A systemic review on pharmacological, phytochemical, toxicological profiles and commercial applications. Res J Pharm Biol Chem Sci. 2013;4:989–1010.
111. Tomar NS, Sharma M, Agarwal RM. Phytochemical analysis of Jatropha curcas L. during different seasons and developmental stages and seedling growth of wheat (Triticum aestivum L) as affected by extracts/leachates of Jatropha curcas L. Physiol Mol Biol Plants. 2015;21(1):83–92.
112. Akbar S. Euphorbia hirta L.; Chamaesyce hirta (L.) Mills. (Euphorbiaceae). Handbook of 200 Medicinal Plants. Cham: Springer; 2020.
113. Ogbulie J, Ogueke C, Okoli IC, Anyanwu BN. Antibacterial activities and toxicological potentials of crude ethanolic extracts of Euphorbia hirta. Afr J Biotechnol. 2007;6(13).
114. Jena J, Gupta A. Ricinus communis linn: A phytopharmacological review. Int J Pharm Pharm Sci. 2012;4:25–9.
115. Singh R, Geetanjali. Phytochemical and pharmacological investigations of Ricinus communis Linn. Algerian J Nat Products. 2015;3:120–9.
116. Zarka M. Chemical composition, antioxidant, cytotoxic and antimicrobial activities of Pimenta racemosa (Mill.) J.W. Moore flower essential oil. J Pharmacogn Phytochem. 2017;6:312–9.
117. Dzib-Reyes EV, García-Sosa K, Simá-Polanco P, Peña-Rodríguez LM. Diterpenoids from the root extract of Chiococca alba. Rev Latinoam Quím. 2012;40(3):123–9.
118. Borges-Argáez R, Medina-Baizabál L, May-Pat F, Peña-Rodríguez LM. A new ent-kaurane from the root extract of Chiococcaalba. Can J Chem. 1997;75(6):801–4.
119. Calixto NO, Pinto MFF, Ramalho SD, Burger MCM, Bobey AF, Young MCM, et al. The Genus Psychotria: Phytochemistry, Chemotaxonomy, Ethnopharmacology and Biological Properties. J Braz Chem Soc. 2016;27(8):1355–78.
120. Singh B, Singh J, Singh JP, Kaur A, Singh N. Phenolic compounds

120. in potato (Solanum tuberosum L.) peel and their health-promoting activities. Int J Food Sci Technol. 2020;55(6):2273–81.
121. Amanpour R, Abbasi-Maleki S, Neyriz-Naghadehi M, Asadi-Samani M. Antibacterial effects of Solanum tuberosum peel ethanol extract in vitro. J Herbmed Pharmacol. 2015;4(2):45–8.
122. Lemus C, Grougnet R, Ellong E, Tian W, Lecsö-Bornet M, Adenet S, et al. Phytochemical study of Capraria biflora L. aerial parts (Scrophulariaceae) from Martinique island (French West Indies). Phytochem Lett. 2015;13.
123. Vasconcellos MC, Montenegro RC, Militão GCG, Fonseca AM, Pessoa ODL, Lemos TLG, et al. Bioactivity of biflorin, a typical o-naphthoquinone isolated from Capraria biflora L. Z Naturforsch C J Biosci. 2005;60(5–6):394–8.
124. Koffuor GA, Ofori-Amoah J, Kyei S, Antwi S, Abokyi S. Anti-tussive, muco-suppressant and expectorant properties, and the safety profile of a hydro-ethanolic extract of Scoparia dulcis. Int J Basic Clin Pharmacol. 2017;3(3):447–53.
125. Riasat-ul-Islam AK, Ansari P, Mousa AY, Haque SMN, Sultana N, Uddin MN, et al. In vitro investigation of antimicrobial, antitumour and DPPH reduction capacity of the methanolic extract of Scoparia dulcis. Microbiol Res J Int. 2015;10(3):1–9.
126. Ahmad I, Zahin M, Aqil F, Hasan S, Khan MSA, Owais M. Bioactive compounds from Punica granatum, Curcuma longa and Zingiber officinale and their therapeutic potential. Drugs Fut. 2008;33(4):329.
127. Bhardwaj KS, Bhardwaj RS, Ranjeet D, Ganesh N. Curcuma longa leaves exhibits a potential antioxidant, antibacterial and immunomodulating properties. Int J Phytomed. 2011;3(2):270–8.
128. Kumar S, Narain U, Tripathi S, Misra K. Syntheses of curcumin bioconjugates and study of their antibacterial activities against beta-lactamase-producing microorganisms. Bioconjug Chem. 2001;12(4):464–9.
129. Sutovska M. Influence of polysaccharides from Aloe vera (Aloe barbadensis Miller, Liliaceae) on mechanically induced cough in cats. Acta Vet Brno. 2010;79(1):51–9.
130. Sahu PK, Giri DD, Singh R, Pandey P, Gupta S, Shrivastava AK, et al. Therapeutic and medicinal uses of Aloe vera: A review. Pharmacol Pharm. 2013; 04(8): 599–610.

131. Mudi SY, Ibrahim H. Activity of Bryophyllum pinnatum S. Kurz extracts on respiratory tract pathogenic bacteria. Bayero J Pure Appl Sci. 2008;1(1):43–8.
132. Ozolua RI, Uwaya DO, Nworgu I, Aigboruan F, Eze YC, Salami EO. Evaluation of the anti-asthmatic and antitussive effects of concurrently administered extracts of Bryophyllum pinnatum and Andrographis paniculata in rodents. J Pharmacy Bioresour. 2017;14(2).
133. Sultana S, Khan A, Safhi MM, Alhazmi HA. Cough suppressant herbal drugs: A review. Int J Pharm Sci Invent. 2016;5(5):15–28.
134. de Araújo AA, Soares LA, Assunção Ferreira MR, de Souza Neto MA, da Silva GR, de Araújo Jr. RF, et al. Quantification of polyphenols and evaluation of antimicrobial, analgesic and anti-inflammatory activities of aqueous and acetone-water extracts of Libidibia ferrea, Parapiptadenia rigida and Psidium guajava. J Ethnopharmacol. 2014;156:88–96.
135. Subramaniam G, Sivasamugham LA, Yew XY. Antibacterial activity of Cymbopogon citratus against clinically important bacteria. S Afr J Chem Eng. 2020;34(1):26–30.
136. Kwon SH, Nam JI, Kim SH, Kim JH, Yoon JH, Kim KS. Kaempferol and quercetin, essential ingredients in Ginkgo biloba extract, inhibit interleukin-1beta-induced MUC5AC gene expression in human airway epithelial cells. Phytother Res. 2009;23(12):1708–12.
137. Potterat O, Hamburger M. Morinda citrifolia (Noni) fruit--phytochemistry, pharmacology, safety. Planta Med. 2007;73(3):191–9.
138. Castillo M, Pascual S, CunhaNune L, Paz Ldl, Canete A. Evaluation of the antimicrobial activity of extracts from leaves and seeds of Morinda citrifolia L. (noni). Rev Cubana Plant Med. 2014;19(4):374–82.
139. Ayunda MN, Zulharmita, Azizah Z, Rivai H. Review of Phytochemical and Pharmacological Activities of Noni (Morinda citrifolia L.). Sch Acad J Pharm 2020; 9:340–346.
140. Hernández-Pérez T, Gómez-García MDR, Valverde ME, Paredes-López O. Capsicum annuum (hot pepper): An ancient Latin-American crop with outstanding bioactive compounds and nutraceutical potential. A review. Compr Rev Food Sci Food Saf. 2020;19(6):2972–93.

141. Bacon K, Boyer R, Denbow C, O'Keefe S, Neilson A, Williams R. Antibacterial activity of jalapeño pepper (Capsicum annuum var. annuum) extract fractions against select foodborne pathogens. Food Sci Nutr. 2017;5(3):730–8.
142. Tang J, Luo K, Li Y, Chen Q, Tang D, Wang D, et al. Capsaicin attenuates LPS-induced inflammatory cytokine production by upregulation of LXRα. Int Immunopharmacol. 2015;28(1):264–9.
143. Wu S, Xiao D. Effect of curcumin on nasal symptoms and airflow in patients with perennial allergic rhinitis. Ann Allergy Asthma Immunol. 2016;117(6):697–702.e1.
144. Birdane L, Cingi C, Muluk NB, San T, Burukoglu D. Evaluation of the efficacy of curcumin in experimentally induced acute sinusitis in rats. Ear Nose Throat J. 2016;95(12):E21–E27.
145. Mao QQ, Xu XY, Cao SY, Gan RY, Corke H, Beta T, et al. Bioactive compounds and bioactivities of ginger (Zingiber officinale Roscoe). Foods. 2019;8(6).
146. Akoachere JF, Ndip RN, Chenwi EB, Ndip LM, Njock TE, Anong DN. Antibacterial effect of Zingiber officinale and Garcinia kola on respiratory tract pathogens. East Afr Med J. 2002;79(11):588–92.
147. Sinan KI, Zengin G, Zheleva-Dimitrova D, Etienne OK, Fawzi Mahomoodally M, Bouyahya A, et al. Qualitative phytochemical fingerprint and network pharmacology investigation of Achyranthes aspera Linn. Extracts. Molecules. 2020;25(8):1973.
148. Mukherjee H, Ojha D, Bag P, Chandel HS, Bhattacharyya S, Chatterjee TK, et al. Anti-herpes virus activities of Achyranthes aspera: An Indian ethnomedicine, and its triterpene acid. Microbiological Research. 2013;168(4):238–44.
149. Choi JG, Lee H, Kim YS, Hwang YH, Oh YC, Lee B, et al. Aloe vera and its components inhibit influenza A virus-induced autophagy and replication. Am J Chin Med. 2019;47(6):1307–24.
150. Borges-Argáez R, Chan-Balan R, Cetina-Montejo L, Ayora-Talavera G, Sansores-Peraza P, Gómez-Carballo J, et al. In vitro evaluation of anthraquinones from Aloe vera (Aloe barbadensis Miller) roots and several derivatives against strains of influenza virus. Ind Crops Prod. 2019;132:468–75.
151. Ogbole O, Akinleye T, Segun P, Faleye T, Adeniji A. In vitro antiviral activity of twenty-seven medicinal plant extracts from Southwest Nigeria against three serotypes of echoviruses. Virol J. 2018;15.

152. Sokolova AS, Yarovaya OI, Semenova MD, Shtro AA, Orshanskaya IR, Zarubaev VV, et al. Synthesis and in vitro study of novel borneol derivatives as potent inhibitors of the influenza A virus. Medchemcomm. 2017;8(5):960–3.
153. Chiang LC, Chang JS, Chen CC, Ng LT, Lin CC. Anti-Herpes simplex virus activity of Bidens pilosa and Houttuynia cordata. Am J Chin Med. 2003;31(3):355–62.
154. Feng L, Zhai Y-Y, Xu J, Cao Y-D, Cheng F-F, Bao B-H, et al. A review on traditional uses, phytochemistry and pharmacology of Eclipta prostrata (L.) L. J Ethnopharmacol. 2019;245:112109.
155. Patel J, Shamim QM, Kumar S, Prasad PU. Phytochemical and pharmacological activities of Eupatorium odoratum L. Research J Pharm and Tech. 2011;4(2):184–8.
156. Roy D, Shaik MM. Toxicology, phytochemistry, bioactive compounds and pharmacology of Parthenium hysterophorus. J Med Plant Stud. 2013;1:126–41.
157. Benassi Zanqueta É, Marques CF, Nocchi SR, Dias Filho BP, Nakamura CV, Ueda-Nakamura T. Parthenolide influences Herpes simplex virus 1 replication in vitro. Intervirology. 2018;61(1):14–22.
158. Hussain H, Al-Harrasi A, Abbas G, Rehman N, Mabood F, Ahmed I, et al. The Genus Pluchea: phytochemistry, traditional uses, and biological activities. Chem Biodivers. 2013;10.
159. Locher C, Witvrouw M, Bethune MD, Burch M, Mower H, Davis H, et al. Antiviral activity of Hawaiian medicinal plants against human immunodeficiency virus Type-1 (HIV-1). Phytomedicine 1996;2(3):259–64.
160. Wijaya S, Nee TK, Jin KT, Hon LK, San LH, Wiart C. Antibacterial and antioxidant activities of Synedrella nodiflora (L.) Gaertn. (Asteraceae). J Complement Integr Med. 2011;8.
161. Amoateng P, Koffuor GA, Sarpong K, Agyapong KO. Free radical scavenging and anti-lipid peroxidative effects of a hydro-ethanolic extract of the whole plant of Synedrella nodiflora (L.) Gaertn (Asteraceae). Free Radic Antiox. 2011;1(3):70–8.
162. Khandagale P, Puri A, Ansari Y, Patil R. Pharmacognostic, physicochemical and phytochemical inverstigation of Caesalpinia bonducella [L.] Roxb. SEED. Int J Pharm Biol Sci. 2018;8:461–8.
163. Al-Snafi A. Pharmacology and medicinal properties of Caesalpinia crista - An overview. Inter J Pharmacy. 2015;5:71–83.

164. Radhakrishnan N, Lam KW, Norhaizan ME. Molecular docking analysis of Carica papaya Linn constituents as antiviral agent. Int Food Res J. 2017;24(4):1819–25.
165. Cryer M, Lane K, Greer M, Cates R, Burt S, Andrus M, et al. Isolation and identification of compounds from Kalanchoe pinnata having human alphaherpesvirus and vaccinia virus antiviral activity. Pharm Biol. 2017;55(1):1586–91.
166. Jia S, Shen M, Zhang F, Xie J. Recent advances in Momordica charantia: functional components and biological activities. Int J Mol Sci. 2017;18(12).
167. Pongthanapisith V, Ikuta K, Puthavathana P, Leelamanit W. Antiviral protein of Momordica charantia L. inhibits different subtypes of Influenza A. Evid Based Complement Alternat Med. 2013;2013:729081.
168. Salatino A, Salatino M, Negri G. Traditional uses, chemistry and pharmacology of Croton species (Euphorbiaceae). J Braz Chem Soc. 2007;18:11–33.
169. Ubillas R. Jolad SD, Bruening RC, Kernan MR, King SR, Sesin DF, et al. SP-303, an antiviral oligomeric proanthocyanidin from the latex of Croton lechleri (Sangre de Drago). Pytomedicine. 1994;1:77.
170. Mao X, Wu L-F, Guo H-L, Chen W-J, Cui Y-P, Qi Q, et al. The genus Phyllanthus: An ethnopharmacological, phytochemical, and pharmacological review. Evid-Based Complement and Altern Med. 2016;2016:7584952.
171. Wang M, Cheng H, Li Y, Meng L, Zhao G, Mai K. Herbs of the genus Phyllanthus in the treatment of chronic hepatitis B: observations with three preparations from different geographic sites. J Lab Clin Med. 1995;126(4):350–2.
172. Yuandani, Ilangkovan M, Jantan I, Mohamad HF, Husain K, Abdul Razak AF. Inhibitory effects of standardized extracts of Phyllanthus amarus and Phyllanthus urinaria and their marker compounds on phagocytic activity of human neutrophils. Evid-based Complement Altern Med. : eCAM, 2013;2013:603634.
173. Bezerra GP, Góis RW, de Brito TS, de Lima FJ, Bandeira MA, Romero NR, et al. Phytochemical study guided by the myorelaxant activity of the crude extract, fractions and constituent from stem bark of Hymenaea courbaril L. J Ethnopharmacol. 2013;149(1):62–9.

174. Cecílio AB, de Faria DB, Oliveira Pde C, Caldas S, de Oliveira DA, Sobral ME, et al. Screening of Brazilian medicinal plants for antiviral activity against rotavirus. J Ethnopharmacol. 2012;141(3):975–81.
175. Yadav JP, Arya V, Yadav S, Panghal M, Kumar S, Dhankhar S. Cassia occidentalis L.: A review on its ethnobotany, phytochemical and pharmacological profile. Fitoterapia. 2009;81:223–30.
176. Vijayalakshmi S, Lingam R, Rajeswari D, Bhagiyalakshmi M. Pharmacological profile of Cassia occidentalis L - A review. Int J Pharm Pharm Sci. 2013;5:29–33.
177. Almeida J, Barbosa J, Cavalcante N, Delange D. A review of the chemical composition and biological activity of Leonotis nepetifolia (Linn.) R. Br. (lion's ear). Rev Cuba Plantas Med. 2018. 2018;23(4).
178. Pushpan R, Nishteswar K, Kumari H. Ethno medicinal claims of Leonotis nepetifolia (L.) R. Br: a review. Int J Res Ayurveda Pharm. 2012;3:783–5.
179. Kumar A, Agarwal K, Maurya AK, Shanker K, Bushra U, Tandon S, et al. Pharmacological and phytochemical evaluation of Ocimum sanctum root extracts for its antiinflammatory, analgesic and antipyretic activities. Pharmacogn Mag. 2015;11(Suppl 1):S217–S24.
180. Chiang LC, Ng LT, Cheng PW, Chiang W, Lin CC. Antiviral activities of extracts and selected pure constituents of Ocimum basilicum. Clin Exp Pharmacol Physiol. 2005;32(10):811–6.
181. Wang Y, Yan W, Chen Q, Huang W, Yang Z, Li X, et al. Inhibition viral RNP and anti-inflammatory activity of coumarins against influenza virus. Biomed Pharmacother. 2017;87:583–8.
182. Hassan MZ, Osman H, Ali MA, Ahsan MJ. Therapeutic potential of coumarins as antiviral agents. Eur J Med Chem. 2016;123:236–55.
183. Arthanari S, Renukadevi P, Vanitha J, Venkateshwaran K, Ganesh M, Clercq ED. Evaluation of antiviral and cytotoxic activities of methanolic extract of Thespesia populnea (Malvaceae) flowers. J Herbs Spices Med Plants. 2011;17(4):386–91.
184. Rangani J, Kumari A, Patel M, Brahmbhatt H, Parida AK. Phytochemical profiling, polyphenol composition, and antioxidant activity of the leaf extract from the medicinal halophyte Thespesia populnea reveal a potential source of bioactive compounds and nutraceuticals. J Food Biochem. 2019;43(2):e12731.
185. Babu SS, Madhuri DB, Ali SL. A pharmacological review of Urena lobata plant. Asian J Pharm Clin Res. 2016;9(2):20–2.

186. Rajtar B, Skalicka-Woźniak K, Świątek Ł, Stec A, Boguszewska A, Polz-Dacewicz M. Antiviral effect of compounds derived from Angelica archangelica L. on Herpes simplex virus-1 and Coxsackievirus B3 infections. Food Chem Toxicol. 2017;109(Pt 2):1026–31.
187. Schwarz S, Sauter D, Wang K, Zhang R, Sun B, Karioti A, et al. Kaempferol derivatives as antiviral drugs against the 3a channel protein of coronavirus. Planta Med. 2014;80(2–3):177–82.
188. Chiamenti L, Silva FP da, Schallemberger K, Demoliner M, Rigotto C, Fleck JD. Cytotoxicity and antiviral activity evaluation of Cymbopogon spp hydroethanolic extracts. Braz J Pharm Sci. 2019;55.
189. Lima IC, Castro RN, Chaves DSA, Ferreira RT, Carvalho MF, Malvar DdC, et al. The folk medicine as tool for discovery of new anti-inflammatory drugs: the example of Spermacoce verticillata. Acta Hortic. 2018;1198(13):67–74.
190. Wu QZ, Zhao DX, Xiang J, Zhang M, Zhang CF, Xu XH. Antitussive, expectorant, and anti-inflammatory activities of four caffeoylquinic acids isolated from Tussilago farfara. Pharm Biol. 2016;54(7):1117–24.
191. Ding Y, Cao Z, Cao L, Ding G, Wang Z, Xiao W. Antiviral activity of chlorogenic acid against influenza A (H1N1/H3N2) virus and its inhibition of neuraminidase. Sci Rep. 2017;7:45723.
192. Izuogu NB, Bello OE, Bello OM. A review on Borreria verticillata: a potential bionematicide, channeling its significant antimicrobial activity against root-knot nematodes. Heliyon. 2020;6(10):e05322.
193. Saleem H, Batool F, Mansoor H, Shahzad-Ul-Hussan S, Saeed M. Inhibition of Dengue virus protease by Eugeniin, Isobiflorin, and Biflorin isolated from the flower buds of Syzygium aromaticum (Cloves). ACS Omega. 2019;4:1525–33.
194. Hayashi K, Niwayama S, Hayashi T, Nago R, Ochiai H, Morita N. In vitro and in vivo antiviral activity of scopadulcic acid B from Scoparia dulcis, Scrophulariaceae, against Herpes simplex virus type 1. Antiviral Res. 1988;9(6):345–54.
195. Liew PM, Yong YK. Stachytarpheta jamaicensis (L.) Vahl: from traditional usage to pharmacological evidence. Evid-based Complement Altern Med. : eCAM. 2016;2016:7842340.
196. Sembiring GF. The effect test of antipyretic infusion of snakeweed

leaf (Stachytarpheta jamaicensis L.) on dove with paracetamol as comparison [master's thesis]. Medan, Indonesia: Health Polytechnic Medan; 2018
197. Woradulayapinij W, Soonthornchareonnon N, Wiwat C. In vitro HIV type 1 reverse transcriptase inhibitory activities of Thai medicinal plants and Canna indica L. rhizomes. J Ethnopharmacol. 2005;101(1–3):84–9.
198. Kumar S, Singh B, Yadav A. Ethanobotany and phytochemistry of Lantana camara L. (Verbenaceae). in: Botanical Leads for Drug Discovery. Singh B, editor. Singapore: Springer; 2020.
199. Hasan R. Antiviral Activity of leaves extract of Lantana camara against the replication of virus A/Puerto Rico/8/34(PR8). Iraqi J Sci. 2017;10:1–8.
200. Braga JM, Pimentel RM, Ferreira CP, Randau KP, Xavier HS. Morphoanatomy, histochemistry and phytochemical screening of Priva lappulacea (L.) Pers. (Verbenaceae). Rev Bras Farmacogn. 2009;19(2b):516–23.
201. Yan H, Ma L, Wang H, Wu S, Huang H, Gu Z, et al. Luteolin decreases the yield of influenza A virus in vitro by interfering with the coat protein I complex expression. J Nat Med. 2019;73(3):487–96.
202. Peng M, Watanabe S, Chan KWK, He Q, Zhao Y, Zhang Z, et al. Luteolin restricts dengue virus replication through inhibition of the proprotein convertase furin. Antiviral Res. 2017;143:176–85.
203. Al-Snafi A. Chemical constituents and pharmacological effects of Asclepias curassavica – a review. Asian J Pharm Res. 2015;5:83–7.
204. Kurdekar RR, Hegde GR, Hebbar SS. Antimicrobial efficacy of Bridelia retusa (Linn.) Spreng and Asclepias curassavica Linn. Indian J Nat Prod Resour. 2012;3(4):589–93.
205. Freitas CDT, Silva RO, Ramos MV, Porfírio C, Farias DF, Sousa JS, et al. Identification, characterization, and antifungal activity of cysteine peptidases from Calotropis procera latex. Phytochemistry. 2020;169:112163.
206. Tomar NS, Sharma M, Agarwal RM. Phytochemical analysis of Jatropha curcas L. during different seasons and developmental stages and seedling growth of wheat (Triticum aestivum L) as affected by extracts/leachates of Jatropha curcas L. Physiol Mol Biol Plants. 2015;21(1):83–92.

207. Saetae D, Suntornsuk W. Antifungal activities of ethanolic extract from Jatropha curcas seed cake. J Microbiol Biotechnol. 2010;20(2):319–24.
208. Rajeh MA Zuraini Z, Sasidharan S, Latha LY, Amutha S. Assessment of Euphorbia hirta L. leaf, flower, stem and root extracts for their antibacterial and antifungal activity and brine shrimp lethality. Molecules. 2010;15(9):6008–18.
209. da Costa MP, Bozinis MCV, Andrade WM, Costa CR, da Silva AL, Alves de Oliveira CM, et al. Antifungal and cytotoxicity activities of the fresh xylem sap of Hymenaea courbaril L. and its major constituent fisetin. BMC Complement Altern Med. 2014;14:245.
210. Idu M, Omonigho SE, Igeleke CL. Preliminary investigation on the phytochemistry and antimicrobial activity of Senna alata L. flower. Pak J Biol Sci. 2007;10(5):806–9.
211. Oladeji O, Adelowo F, Oluyori A, Bankole D. Ethnobotanical description and biological activities of Senna alata. Evid-J Evid Based Complement Alternat Med. 2020;2020:1–12.
212. Bento EB, Júnior FEB, de Oliveira DR, Fernandes CN, de Araújo Delmondes G, Cesário F, et al. Antiulcerogenic activity of the hydroalcoholic extract of leaves of Annona muricata Linnaeus in mice. Saudi J Biol Sci. 2018;25(4):609–21.
213. Siqueira ADMO, Moreira ACCG, Melo EDA, Stamford TCM, Stamford TLM. Dietary fibre content, phenolic compounds and antioxidant activity in soursops (Annona muricata L.). Rev Bras Frutic. 2015;37:1020–6.
214. Hwang DY. Therapeutic role of natural products containing tannin for treatment of constipation. Mózsik G, editor: Intech.; 2019.
215. Ashafa AOT, Sunmonu T, Abass A, Ogbe A. Laxative potential of the ethanolic leaf extract of Aloe vera (L.) Burm. f. in Wistar rats with loperamide-induced constipation. J Nat Pharm. 2011;2(3):158.216. Sánchez M, González-Burgos E, Iglesias I, Gómez-Serranillos MP. Pharmacological update properties of Aloe vera and its major active constituents. Molecules. 2020;25(6).
217. Khedmat H, Karbasi A, Amini M, Aghaei A, Taheri S. Aloe vera in treatment of refractory irritable bowel syndrome: Trial on Iranian patients. J Res Med Sci. 2013;18(8):732.
218. Chukwuka KS, Iwuagwu M, Uka UN. Evaluation of nutritional

components of Carica papaya L. at different stages of ripenening. IOSR J Pharm and Biol Sci. 2013;6(4):13–6.
219. Duangjai A, Nuengchamnong N, Lee L-H, Goh B-H, Saokaew S, Suphrom N. Characterisation of an extract and fractions of Azadirachta indica flower on cholesterol lowering property and intestinal motility. Nat Prod Res. 2019;33(10):1491–4.
220. Bennett A, Stamford IF, Tavares IA, Jacobs S, Capasso F, Mascolo N, et al. The biological activity of eugenol, a major constituent of nutmeg (Myristica fragrans): studies on prostaglandins, the intestine and other tissues. Phytother Res. 1988;2(3):124–30.
221. Paul S, Hwang JK, Kim HY, Jeon WK, Chung C, Han JS. Multiple biological properties of macelignan and its pharmacological implications. Arch Pharm Res. 2013;36(3):264–72.
222. Ali SM, Khan AA, Ahmed I, Musaddiq M, Ahmed KS, Polasa H, et al. Antimicrobial activities of eugenol and cinnamaldehyde against the human gastric pathogen Helicobacter pylori. Ann Clin Microbiol Antimicrob. 2005;4:20.
223. Barrowman JA, Bennett A, Hillenbrand P, Rolles K, Pollock DJ, Wright JT. Diarrhoeae in thyroid medullary carcinoma: role of prostaglandins and therapeutic effect of nutmeg. Br Med J. 1975;3(5974):11–2.
224. Francisco V, Figueirinha A, Costa G, Liberal J, Lopes MC, García-Rodríguez C, et al. Chemical characterization and anti-inflammatory activity of luteolin glycosides isolated from lemongrass. J Funct Foods. 2014;10:436–43.
225. Devi RC, Sim SM, Ismail R. Spasmolytic effect of citral and extracts of Cymbopogon citratus on isolated rabbit ileum. J Smooth Muscle Res. 2011;47(5):143–56.
226. Christian E O, Okwesili Fc N, Parker E J, Okechukwu Pc U. Acute toxicity investigation and anti-diarrhoeal effect of the chloroform-methanol extract of the leaves of Persea americana. Iran J Pharm Res. 2014;13(2):651–8.
227. Boiko Y, Kravchenko I, Shandra A, Boiko I. Extraction, identification and anti-inflammatory activity of carotenoids out of Capsicum anuum L. J Herbmed Pharmacol. 2017;6(1):10–5.
228. Bortolotti M, Porta S. Effect of red pepper on symptoms of irritable bowel syndrome: preliminary study. Dig Dis Sci. 2011;56(11):3288–95.

229. Labban L. Medicinal and pharmacological properties of turmeric (Curcuma longa): a review. Int J Pharm Biomed Sci. 2014;5(1):17–23.
230. Pertz HH, Lehmann J, Roth-Ehrang R, Elz S. Effects of ginger constituents on the gastrointestinal tract: role of cholinergic M3 and serotonergic 5-HT3 and 5-HT4 receptors. Planta Med. 2011;77(10):973–8.
231. Barkat MQ, Mahmood HK. Phytochemical and antioxidant screening Of Zingiber officinale, Piper nigrum, Rutag raveolanes and Carum carvi and their effect on gastrointestinal tract activity. Matrix Sci Medica. 2018;2(1):9–13.
232. Anyasor GN, Moses N, Kale O. Hepatoprotective and hematological effects of Justicia secunda Vahl leaves on carbon tetrachloride induced toxicity in rats. Biotech Histochem. 2020;95(5):349–59.
233. Moosavian SP, Paknahad Z, Habibagahi Z, Maracy M. The effects of garlic (Allium sativum) supplementation on inflammatory biomarkers, fatigue, and clinical symptoms in patients with active rheumatoid arthritis: A randomized, double-blind, placebo-controlled trial. Phytother Res. 2020;34(11):2953–62.
234. Hedaya R. Five herbs plus thiamine reduce pain and improve functional mobility in patients with pain: A pilot study. Altern Ther Health Med. 2017;23(1):14–9.
235. Badgujar SB, Patel VV, Bandivdekar AH. Foeniculum vulgare Mill: a review of its botany, phytochemistry, pharmacology, contemporary application, and toxicology. Biomed Res Int. 2014;2014:842674-.
236. Khan MS, Hamid A, Akram M, Mustafa SB, Sami A, Shah SMA, et al. Antipyretic potential of herbal coded formulation (Pyrexol). Pak J Pharm Sci. 2017;30(1):195–8.
237. Yousofi A, Daneshmandi S, Soleimani N, Bagheri K, Karimi MH. Immunomodulatory effect of parsley (Petroselinum crispum) essential oil on immune cells: mitogen-activated splenocytes and peritoneal macrophages. Immunopharmacol Immunotoxicol. 2012;34(2):303–8.
238. Aydin G, Kaya E. A review: Momordica charantia L.'s biological active components and its potential use in traditional therapies. Int J Tradit Compleme Med Res. 2020;1(2):79–95.
239. M. Knowlton W, D. McKemy D. TRPM8: From cold to cancer, peppermint to pain. Curr Pharm Biotechnol. 2011;12(1):68–77.

240. Ilango K, Maharajan G, Narasimhan S. Anti-nociceptive and anti-inflammatory activities of Azadirachta indica fruit skin extract and its isolated constituent azadiradione. Nat Prod Res. 2013;27(16):1463–7.
241. Srivastava S, Agrawal B, Kumar A, Pandey A. Phytochemicals of Azadirachta indica source of active medicinal constituent used for cure of various diseases: a review. J Sci Res. 2020;64:285–90.
242. Mehwish HM, Riaz Rajoka MS, Xiong Y, Zheng K, Xiao H, Anjin T, et al. Moringa oleifera: a functional food and its potential immunomodulatory effects. Food Rev Int. 2020:1–20.
243. Boukhatem MN, Ferhat MA, Kameli A, Saidi F, Kebir HT. Lemon grass (Cymbopogon citratus) essential oil as a potent anti-inflammatory and antifungal drugs. Libyan J Med. 2014;9:25431.
244. Mendes Hacke AC, Miyoshi E, Marques JA, Pereira RP. Anxiolytic properties of Cymbopogon citratus (DC.) stapf extract, essential oil and its constituents in zebrafish (Danio rerio). J Ethnopharmacol. 2020;260:113036.
245. Zige DV, Ohimain E. Efficacy of Cymbopogon citratus and Carica papaya used in the traditional treatment of enteric fever against Salmonella in Bayelsa State, Nigeria. EC Microbiol 2017; 6: 80–88.
246. Chen Z, Quan L, Zhou H, Zhao Y, Chen P, Hu L, et al. Screening of active fractions from Curcuma Longa Radix isolated by HPLC and GC-MS for promotion of blood circulation and relief of pain. J Ethnopharmacol. 2019;234:68–75.
247. Black CD, Herring MP, Hurley DJ, O'Connor PJ. Ginger (Zingiber officinale) reduces muscle pain caused by eccentric exercise. J Pain. 2010;11(9):894–903.
248. Wu HC, Horng CT, Tsai SC, Lee YL, Hsu SC, Tsai YJ, et al. Relaxant and vasoprotective effects of ginger extracts on porcine coronary arteries. Int J Mol Med. 2018;41(4):2420–8.
249. Yasir M, Das S, Kharya MD. The phytochemical and pharmacological profile of Persea americana Mill. Pharmacogn Rev. 2010 Jan;4(7):77–84. doi: 10.4103/0973-7847.65332. PMID: 22228945; PMCID:PMC3249906.
250. Thabet AA, Moghannem S, Ayoub IM, Youssef FS, Al Sayed E, Singab ANB. GC/MS profiling of essential oils from Bontia daphnoides L., chemometric discrimination, isolation of dehydroepingaione and

evaluation of antiviral activity. Sci Rep. 2022 Oct 21;12(1):17707. doi:10.1038/s41598-022-22174-4. PMID: 36271233; PMCID: PMC9587025.

251. Conserva LM, Ferreira JC Jr. Borreria and Spermacoce species (Rubiaceae): A review of their ethnomedicinal properties, chemical constituents, and biological activities. Pharmacogn Rev. 2012 Jan;6(11):46-55. doi: 10.4103/0973-7847.95866. PMID: 22654404; PMCID: PMC3358967.

252. Aćimović M, Jeremić K, Salaj N, Gavarić N, Kiprovski B, Sikora V, Zeremski T. Marrubium vulgare L.: A Phytochemical and Pharmacological Overview. Molecules. 2020 Jun 24;25(12):2898. doi: 10.3390/molecules25122898. PMID: 32599693;PMCID: PMC7355696.

253. Paikra BK, Dhongade HKJ, Gidwani B. Phytochemistry and Pharmacology of Moringa oleifera Lam. J Pharmacopuncture. 2017 Sep;20(3):194–200. doi: 10.3831/KPI.2017.20.022. Epub 2017 Sep 30. PMID: 30087795; PMCID:PMC5633671.

254. Patel, Jitendra & Shamim, Q.M. & Kumar, Shiv & Prasad, P.U. (2011). Phytochemical and pharmacological activities of Eupatorium odoratum L. *Research Journal of Pharmacy and Technology*. 4. 184–188.

255. Cervantes-Ceballos L, Sánchez-Hoyos J, Sanchez-Hoyos F, Torres-Niño E, Mercado-Camargo J, Echeverry-Gómez A, Jotty Arroyo K, Del Olmo-Fernández E, Gómez-Estrada H. An Overview of Genus Malachra L.-Ethnobotany, Phytochemistry, and Pharmacological Activity. Plants (Basel). 2022 Oct 22;11(21):2808. doi: 10.3390/plants11212808. PMID: 36365260; PMCID: PMC9657199.

256. Ekpenyong CE, Akpan E, Nyoh A. Ethnopharmacology, phytochemistry, and biological activities of Cymbopogon citratus (DC.) Stapf extracts. Chin J Nat Med. 2015 May;13(5):321–37. doi: 10.1016/S1875-5364(15)30023-6. PMID: 25986281.

257. Bahramsoltani R, Ahmadian R, Daglia M, Rahimi R. Petroselinum crispum (Mill.) Fuss (Parsley): An Updated Review of the Traditional Uses, Phytochemistry, and Pharmacology. J Agric Food Chem. 2024 Jan 17;72(2):956-972. doi: 10.1021/acs.jafc.3c06429. Epub 2024 Jan 8. PMID: 38189231.

258. Lima EB, Sousa CN, Meneses LN, Ximenes NC, Santos Júnior MA, Vasconcelos GS, Lima NB, Patrocínio MC, Macedo D, Vasconcelos

SM. Cocos nucifera (L.) (Arecaceae): A phytochemical and pharmacological review. Braz J Med Biol Res. 2015 Nov;48(11):953–64. doi: 10.1590/1414-31X20154773. Epub 2015 Aug 18. PMID: 26292222; PMCID: PMC4671521.

3

Plant Nomenclature, Chemistry and Appraisal of Practices in Barbados

PLANT NOMENCLATURE

THE SCIENTIFIC NAMING OF PLANTS is governed by a set of rules and recommendations established as the International Code of Nomenclature for Algae, Fungi and Plants. Prior to 2011, this code was known as the International Code of Botanical Nomenclature (ICBN). In its current form, it governs the naming of all organisms traditionally treated as algae, fungi or plants, whether fossil or fossil related, including blue-green algae (Cyanobacteria), chytrids, oomycetes, slime, moulds, and photosynthetic protists with their taxonomically related non-photosynthetic groups (excluding Microsporidia) (62). Within the code, each plant belongs to an infinite number of Latinized taxa. A taxon (plural taxa) is a biological unit of classification arranged in a hierarchical ranking system from kingdom to species or sub-species. The sequence of ranks in descending order are kingdom, division or phylum, class, order, family, genus and species. The botanical name of a plant is a combination of the genus and species however, this rule doesn't exclude specific species which may be named with ranks higher than genus.

The folklore naming of plants does not appear to be governed by any formal code and the use of terminology is generally colloquial in the assignment of names. The common names of plants, especially of medicinal plants, are rooted in the cultural traditions and language of the society in which the plants are found. These names were ascribed to plants long before the scientific system for naming plants was established. The common name is used mainly as an alternative to the scientific name by lay individuals within a given jurisdiction and may be bound geographically or culturally or sometimes both. These names are generally interpreted figuratively and are literal seldomly according to the dictionaries of the language of the country of origin (28, 63). Some common names may appear to be quite universal, for example, Noni, Lemon grass/Fever grass, Ginger and Garlic, and is related to the wide use of the plant derived through cultural syncretism. Most plants in the Caribbean are not confined to any one Caribbean territory as the inhabitants of the Caribbean inclusive of the indigenous people, West Africans, Europeans, and indentured servants migrated throughout the region with their cultures and practices. Barbados has been known to have 650–700 species of plants and only two are considered endemic to the island, emphasising this point. Most of the plant species on the island can be found in other tropical climate regions. Due to the lack of a formal systematic approach to the naming of plants colloquially, the following are potential issues that can arise:

1. Same plants have different common names, for example: Spanish Needles, Duppy Needles, Monkey Needles (*Bidens pilosa*)
2. Common names can change with the evolution of cultures
3. A single common name can refer to different species of the same genus for example Seed-Under-Leaf (*Phyllanthus niruri* and *Phyllanthus amarus*)

THE CHEMICAL PROFILING OF THE MEDICINAL PLANTS

Recent molecular approaches in phylogeny allows plants to be differentiated into about 500 plant families (20). Former approaches in phylogeny were based on the plants' phenotypes inclusive of the plant morphology and their chemical profile. The chemical profile provides an overview of the chemical constituents of the plant. Chemical constituents of plants with discrete bioactivities towards animal biochemistry and metabolism are categorised as phytochemicals (64). The phytochemicals are commonly termed secondary metabolites in contrast to compounds termed primary metabolites which are essential for plant growth and development. These secondary metabolites are important in facilitating the plant's interactions with the abiotic and biotic environment. They fulfil important roles such as defence against herbivores and pathogens, produce flower pigments to attract pollinators, produce hormones and other or signal molecules, and are also used by humans as condiments, pigments and for health related effects (64, 65). The four major classifications of phytochemicals based on their biosynthetic origin include alkaloids, phenylpropanoids, polyketides and terpenoids.

Alkaloids represent one of the most medically relevant groups of phytochemicals and are defined as heterocyclic nitrogen compounds biosynthesized from amino acids. Examples of drugs derived from alkaloids include: atropine, an anticholinergic; caffeine, a stimulant; cocaine, local anaesthetic and stimulant; vincristine (Vinca alkaloid), an anticancer drug; and scopolamine, an anticholinergic. (65). Phenylpropanoids are a diverse group of phytochemicals and are synthesised from primary metabolites, phenylalanine or tyrosine amino acids. They can be further classified into flavonoids, lignin, phenolic acids, stilbenes and coumarins (66, 67). These compounds are known for their antioxidant effects (64). Polyketides are derived from a precursor molecule consisting of a chain of alternating ketone (or reduced forms of a ketone) and methylene groups. They are structurally diverse and possess a wide range of bioactivities. The antibiotic, tetracycline is an example of polyketides (68). Terpenoids, otherwise called terpenes or isoprenoids, are considered the largest group of phytochemicals, and are derived from five-carbon isoprene units. They are further classified as hemiterpenes, monoterpenes, sesquiterpenes, diterpenes, triterpenes, tetraterpenes and polyterpenes. The antimalarial drug artemisinin is a sesquiterpene and the anticancer drug paclitaxel is a diterpene (65).

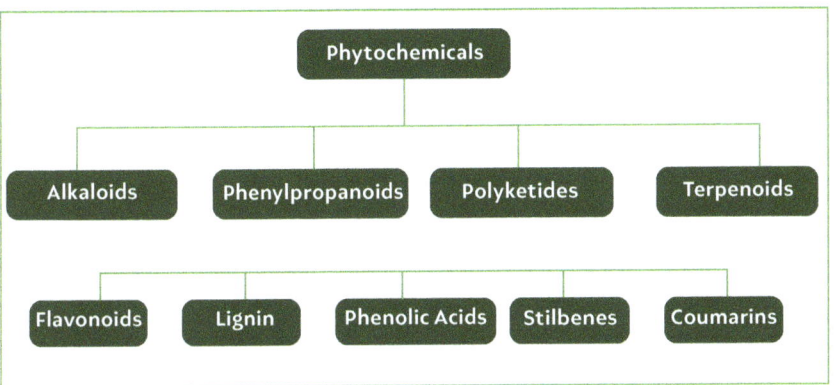

Figure 3.1: Classification of Phytochemicals (Secondary Metabolites) in Plants (65)

Phytochemicals have been the foundation for drug discovery and modern medicine. Recent trends suggest that it is becoming more difficult to explore naturally derived plant compounds for drug discovery. Variations in legal frameworks have caused inertia on obtaining intellectual property rights for unmodified natural products in countries that do not grant patents for naturally occurring compounds in their original form. Also, biopiracy of the biodiversity rich tropical countries has been an ongoing problem with no sensible solution so far. The United Nations 1992 Convention on Biological Biodiversity and the Nagoya Protocol have imposed some limitations on profitability of exploring natural based compounds due to the legal requirement for benefit sharing with the countries from which the biological material originate. Historically, there have always been issues with bioactivity-guided isolation and the complexity of the compounds' size and polarity which impact their application as medicines (69). Synthetic compounds or analogues of natural based compounds are used as alternatives to stem the issues highlighted with the harvesting and the commercial scale-up of medicinal compounds from plants.

Phytochemicals are extracted by various solvent media which transcends the polarity series prior to characterisation. Most of the plant preparations listed in chapter 2 are hot infusions and decoctions to make teas or percolation with ethanol-based liquor to make tinctures. Other extraction processes inclusive of the use of the Soxhlet, Steam

Distillation and Supercritical Carbon Dioxide (CO2) techniques must be pursued in the laboratory or industrial environments. The genesis of the phytochemicals and their physiochemical properties are important for the isolation of the medicinal or other bioactivities of the plant. Therefore, extraction methods should be aligned with the phytochemical groups and their physiochemical properties. Close to 100% of the entries identified for the treatment of communicable and non-communicable diseases in the review in chapter 2 contain pharmacologically active phytochemicals. In some cases, the chemical profiling of the plants was not able to identify specific bioactive compounds but could identify the phytochemical group likely to be associated with the medicinal effect(s). Some of these phytochemical groups were identified under the categories outlined in figure 3.1. Many of these phytochemical groups, such as the flavonoids, are known generally to have bioactivity inclusive of antioxidant, antimicrobial properties and enzyme inhibition (64, 70).

Some studies reported preliminary investigations with the extracts of the plants and not the specific bioactive ingredient. In such cases, it is difficult to associate the bioactivity of the extract with any specific chemical constituent without conducting bioactivity-guided isolation of the compounds. Additional chemical and pharmacological investigations are in progress on these plants to identify the bioactive constituents which are related to the specific uses of the plant.

APPRAISAL OF THE REPORTED BIOACTIVITY

The most recent ethnopharmacological study done in a rural district in St. John, Barbados identified a total of 29 medicinal applications cited across 69 different plant species and 39 families (42). The most popular species among rural respondents (irrespective of use) were *Pimenta racemosa* (Mill.) J.W. Moore (Bay Leaf), *Momordica charantia* L. (Cerasee), *Zingiber officinale* Roscoe (Ginger) and *Annona muricata* L. (Soursop) (42). The findings on the use of botanical medicines in this study also suggest a rural-urban divide on the retention of indigenous and ancestral practices as 75% of the rural respondents reported using medicinal plants. Earlier ethnopharmacological studies across the island of Barbados suggested that approximately a third (33.3%) of the population use botanical medicines (40, 41).

Traditional uses of medicinal plants in Barbados have been mainly aligned with the treatment of tropical and systemic infectious diseases. Most of these practices are aligned with the disease profile of the Caribbean during the seventeenth to twentieth centuries (11) when infectious conditions were more prevalent. In the twenty-first century, urbanisation and an improved human development index in Barbados have contributed to the development of sedentary lifestyles and diseases. Moreover, the use of antibiotics and vaccines have led to a reduction in the prevalence in communicable diseases. The 2015 Health of the Nation study in Barbados found that 1 in 10 adults has a Chronic Noncommunicable Disease (15). These diseases account for eight of the ten causes of death in Barbados in 2019 (9). This change in the disease profile has led to the expansion of the use of medicinal plants to treat these diseases.

In chapter 2, almost all plant entries identified as the treatment options for communicable and non-communicable diseases, and other ailments contain pharmacologically active phytochemicals. Similarly, almost all of the plant entries reported bioactivities consistent with their reported use. Further analysis of these findings outlines that of the medicinal plant entries for the treatment of non-communicable diseases, almost all identified pharmacological active compounds in these plants with accompanying studies reporting bioactivities consistent with their reported use. Similarly for communicable conditions, most of the medicinal plant entries identified pharmacologically active compounds in the plants, with studies reporting bioactivities consistent with their reported use. For conditions which were not classified as communicable and non-communicable, close to 100% of the plant entries identified pharmacologically active compounds, with studies reporting activities consistent with their reported use. This confirms that more scientific information supporting the traditional uses of a number of locally used medicinal plants have been identified compared to previously published data in the first edition of *Medicinal Plants of Barbados*. In the first edition, 61% of the plant entries for the treatment of communicable and non-communicable diseases had pharmacologically active compounds identified. Fifty-one per cent of these entries had studies reporting activities consistent with the reported use of the plants.

Table 3.1 outlines some plants which are used for medicinal purposes and scientific literature highlighting bioactivities consistent to their traditional uses. More details on the scientific studies supporting the use of the plants can be found in chapter 2.

Table 3.1: Reported Bioactivities of Popularly Used Medicinal Plants

Major Disease Categories	Plant Species (Common Name)	Validation of Potential Use
Bacterial Infections	*Bidens pilosa* (Duppy Needles/ Monkey Needles/ Spanish Needles)	Antibacterial effects of phytochemicals were validated by an ethanolic extract which has a wide spectrum of antibacterial activity. (71)
	Jatropha curcas (Physic Nut)	Studies reported in *Phorbol Esters: Structure, Biological Activity, and Toxicity in Animals* (Goel et al. 2007); validated the plant's anti-infective effect. (72) The antimicrobial activity and phytochemical screening of the extracts of stem bark from *Jatropha curcas* was also reported. (73)
Viral Infections	*Pluchea carolinensis* (Cure-For-All)	Antiviral activity of triterpenoids found in the plant on Herpes simplex virus-infected cells *in vitro* has been reported. (74)
	Phyllanthus amarus (Seed-Under-Leaf)	*Phyllanthus amarus* suppresses hepatitis B virus by interrupting interactions between HBV enhancer I and cellular transcription factors. (75)
Fungal Infections	*Jatropha curcas* (Physic Nut)	Antifungal activities of the ethanolic extract from *Jatropha curcas* seed cake have been reported. (76)
	Hymenaea courbaril (Locust Tree/Stinking Toe Tree)	Antifungal terpenoid, caryophyllene epoxide, defends a neotropical tree (Hymenaea) against attack by fungus-growing ants. (77)

Table 3.1 continues

Major Disease Categories	Plant Species (Common Name)	Validation of Potential Use
Cardiovascular Conditions (for example hypertension and atherosclerosis)	*Peperomia pellucida* (Shine Bush)	(i) Significant anti-hypercholesterolemia effects, reducing total cholesterol and LDL while increasing HDL levels. (78) (ii) Plant extract shown to increase inhibitory effect of endogenous ACE inhibitors, thus helping to lower blood pressure; a flavonoid inhibitor of ACE was also identified in the plant extract. (79, 80) (iii) Intravenous administration of an extract with cardiac glycosides caused reductions in systolic and diastolic blood pressure, and mean arterial pressure. (81)
Diabetes	*Tecoma stans* (Christmas hope, Elder Bush)	(i) Rutin-rich flavonoid extract had potent postprandial anti-hyperglycaemic effects due to α-glucosidase inhibition; alkaloid-rich extract significantly reduced blood glucose levels. (82) (ii) Flavonoids & β-sitosterol shown to induce adipogenesis, improve glucose uptake in adipocytes, improve translocation of Glucose Transporter (GLUT) 2 and 4, and decrease insulin resistance. (83, 84)
	Phyllanthus niruri (Seed-Under-Leaf)	(i) Effective anti-hyperglycaemic activity demonstrated by significantly reducing fasting blood glucose levels and suppressing postprandial rise in blood glucose in rats. (85) (ii) Extract neutralised Reactive Oxygen Species (ROS) and attenuated endogenous antioxidant enzymes to normal levels. (86)

Table 3.1 continues

Major Disease Categories	Plant Species (Common Name)	Validation of Potential Use
Cancer	Phyllanthus amarus (Seed-Under-Leaf)	Plant extract exhibited anti-metastatic activity and inhibited breast and lung carcinoma cell growth; effectively reducing invasion, migration, and adhesion of both cell types and deemed capable of inducing apoptosis. (87)
	Peperomia pellucida	(i) Plant extract displayed significant cytotoxic activity against human cervical cancer and hepatic carcinoma cell lines. (88) (ii) Plant extract inhibited growth of human promyelocytic leukaemia, breast cancer, and cervical cancer cells. (89)
	Physalis angulata (Cow Pops, Poppers)	(i) Extract significantly inhibited metastasis and proliferation of oral cancer cells. (90) (ii) Novel compounds identified that showed significant cytotoxic activities on three human cancer cell lines. (91, 92)
	Catharanthus roseus (Madagascar Periwinkle)	Has Vinca alkaloids Vincristine & Vinblastine (USFDA anticancer drug compounds)
Neurodegenerative Diseases	Synedrella nodiflora	Leaf extract produced cerebroprotective effects in global cerebral ischemia in rats and reduced hyperlocomotion and neuronal damage. (93)

As observed in chapter 2, a limited number of plants showed similar bioactive compounds in their phytochemical profiles to approved active pharmaceutical ingredients used in conventional pharmacotherapy of illnesses and conditions. This finding may be due to the vast number of drug candidates which are still undergoing research but are yet to be approved by drug regulatory bodies e.g. USFDA or European Medicine Authority (EMA), or the lack of studies on phytochemicals derived from medicinal plants used extensively in the Caribbean. The latter may be related to issues of intellectual property laws in Caribbean jurisdictions, issues of benefit sharing as required under the Nagoya Protocol and limitations of the use of plant-based compounds in drug discovery mentioned earlier. Examples of drug compounds approved by drug regulatory authorities for similar indications to their derived plant sources are the vinca alkaloids, vincristine and vinblastine, from the plant *Catharanthus roseus* in the botanical family Apocynaceae. These two compounds are approved anticancer agents. To the contrary, some of the approved drug compounds with similar chemical structure to compounds found in the chemical profile of plants were identified as treatment options for other illnesses not indicated by a local folklore claim. For example, the plant compound parthenolide, isolated from the plant *Parthenium hysterophorus*, was found to be an effective antiviral compound specifically against the Herpes simplex virus -1. However, this compound has been used in a phase I dose escalation clinical trial of Feverfew (a plant extract with parthenolide but isolated from the plant *Tanacetum parthenium*) in patients with cancer (94). Chapter 2 outlines the ethnobotanical use of *Parthenium hysterophorus* as an antiviral agent. This evidence indicates that some bioactive plant compounds may have multiple uses for the treatment of diseases, both communicable and non-communicable conditions. Some antiviral agents have been shown to have anticancer chemotherapeutic effects, such as interferon-alpha-2a. The rationale for the dual purposes is that the mechanism of action of these compounds as an anti-infective agent may be related to the compound's mechanism of action as an anti-cancer agent with anti-metabolite effects or having a direct effect on nucleic acid synthesis and processing.

In cases where an active pharmaceutical ingredient was not found to be associated with a bioactive compound from a plant, literature sources were used to identify a phytochemical being evaluated for the reported traditional use. The review of the scientific literature also showed that some plants were tested for conditions other than those which were identified for the local use of medicinal plants. This occurrence points to the vast number of phytochemicals in plants. It could also be linked to the variety of medicinal uses of the same plant in different territories. These other uses were not reported, as the purpose of this investigation was to validate the local uses of medicinal plants.

BEST PRACTICES WHEN CONSIDERING PLANT BASED MEDICINES

The use of medicinal plants for the treatment of diseases is universal according to the World Health Organisation with approximately 70–90% or more of the world's population using plants for some part of their primary healthcare (45, 46, 95). While the reports of the use of plants across the island of Barbados for medicinal purposes, 33.3%, is significantly lower (40), it is important to highlight best practices for the use of plant-based medicines in their natural and commodified forms. These best practices are related to standardisation, establishing efficacy and safety, and understanding the concept of drug-herb interactions.

Standardisation and Dosages

Herbs and other plants used for medicinal purposes can be harvested or procured for use; in their natural state (fresh); minimally processed as dried flowers, fruits, leaves, stems and roots; lightly commodified as oils, teas, and tinctures; and extensively commodified, as dietary supplements and nutraceuticals. All forms may vary significantly in the phytochemicals which contribute to the medicinal effect. Even different batches of the same plant or product from the same planter/producer may differ in quantity and quality of phytochemicals which will influence its related efficacy due to the harvesting period, location of the cultivation of the plant, method of preparation and administration route (96). Within conventional medical disciplines such as pharmacology and by extension, pharmacotherapeutics, the concept of a dose-response relationship is used for the therapeutic dosing of a drug or a medicinal substance. The concept outlines that a given dose of the drug or medicine will produce a physiological effect at a given magnitude for a specified period. This effect can be observed within a physiological system and will increase incrementally with the dose of the drug until the response is at a maximum level. This is described as a *graded dose-response* relationship. The other dose-response relationship describes the response of a given sample of a population to a dose of a drug or medicine which can also increase to a maximum and is described as a *quantal dose-response* relationship (26). The latter is used in deciphering the safety of drugs and medicines. A dose of a medicine is a uniform quantity designated by its weight or weight by volume in a standardised solution of a medicine linked to the desired therapeutic effect and safety in a patient (97). Several factors are considered in ascertaining a dose of a medicine including the bioactivity and the chemical properties of substances in the medicine, the route of administration, the distribution of the medicinal substance in the body and the elimination of the medicine from the body. Over centuries, traditional healing practices established dosages by repeated observations from practitioners in 'uncontrolled' natural but scientific settings. This can be contrasted to westernised treatment approaches, where medicines and doses were established from 'controlled' scientific experiments (28, 39, 97). Traditional approaches have undergone continuous transformation due to syncretism to align with westernised approaches (28). For example, the practice of making teas from plants with medicinal benefits have been redesigned and branded into a household approach of making teas by hot infusion of dried plant material (2.5 grams) in a sachet with a cup (about 240 millilitres) of boiling water.

Establishing Efficacy and Safety

The therapeutic dosing of a drug is adjudicated by its efficacy and safety. Efficacy is used interchangeably with effectiveness when describing the therapeutic ability of a medicine. From a biochemical viewpoint, efficacy is described as the response elicited when a drug interacts with its biological target central to the disease (26). The safety of medicines is construed in the limiting of drug toxicity. Drug toxicity arises from four main mechanisms: i) inappropriate activation or inhibition of the intended drug targets or unintended drug targets ii) formation of a toxic metabolite of the drug; iii) inappropriate immune responses and iv) idiosyncratic drug responses (98). All the mechanisms except the last are self-explanatory. Idiosyncratic responses are rare adverse effects linked to unique individual genetic differences in response to drugs caused primarily by variations in metabolism or immune system response (26). Plant compounds are natural, but this does not prevent them from being toxic for human use. As mentioned in the section, *The Chemical Profiling of Medicinal Plants*, the secondary metabolites of plants are not only medicinal but facilitate the abiotic and biotic interaction of the plant with its environment. This includes roles such as defence against herbivores and pathogens (64, 65). Uncontrolled and controlled experimental approaches in traditional and westernised medicine respectively have facilitated our understanding of toxicity and the safe use of medicines. Traditional practitioners would use indigenous scientific methods to observe the interaction of animals, inclusive of birds and mammals, and the plants to draw inferences on safety of the plants or their extracts. Even with the elaborate background on the use of plants as medicines as precursors to conventional drugs and the extensive use of plants as medicines globally, many medicinal plants and products have yet to be subjected to the same rigorous efficacy and safety trials as conventional drugs (99). In contrast to traditional medicine, westernised approaches for establishing the efficacy and safety of a medicine have been confined to controlled preclinical and clinical development of drugs and usually identifies a single drug compound as opposed to the complementary (opposing or synergistic) compounds that would be there in plant preparations. More so, most of the currently available studies inclusive of systematic reviews investigating the uses of plant-based preparations focus extensively on commodified products, which are marketed and widely used in westernised countries. However, many of the plants used in Caribbean folk medicine seem to be assessed for bioactivities consistent with their reported uses but hardly investigated to establish efficacy and safety for mainstream medical applications (51). The issue of efficacy and safety is heightened locally by many Barbadians who will simply self-diagnose and try to cure themselves instead of seeing a physician.

Concomitant use of Herbal Remedies and Drugs, Polypharmacy and Drug Interactions

A common practice among some users of traditional medicine is the use of multiple medicines, inclusive of herbal medicines, leading to practices of polypharmacy (100). Polypharmacy is the simultaneous use of multiple drugs or medicinal substances, (often more than 5) for therapy. In Barbados and other Caribbean jurisdictions, there are reports of patients using plant-based medicines concomitantly with conventional medicine especially for the management of chronic Non-communicable Diseases (cNCDs). (40, 47, 50, 100). This practice is potentially problematic however, has been corroborated with the widespread use of plant-based medicines globally. This finding also suggests a positive perception of the use of medicinal plants among populations with indigenous or culturally derived traditional practices (45, 56).

Polypharmacy is normally monitored in the clinical (in-patient) and out-patient settings because of the possibilities of adverse drug reactions related to drug interactions. A drug interaction occurs when the response of a patient to a drug is changed by the presence of another drug, food, drink or by some environmental chemical agent (26). The interactions may increase or decrease the pharmacological and toxicological effects of the drug or medicinal substance. The chemical constituents from plant-based remedies may interfere with the effects of conventional drugs or *vice versa* by pharmacokinetic or pharmacodynamic interactions when herbal products are used concomitantly with drugs. These interactions can also occur between two plant-based compounds when herbal products are used together. Pharmacokinetic interactions are those which can affect the processes by which drugs or phytochemicals are absorbed, distributed, metabolised, and excreted. Interactions which interfere with the activity of the cytochrome P 450 and conjugating enzymes of the liver are well documented to increase or decrease efficacy of other medicines by enzyme inhibition or induction (increased de nova synthesis of liver isozymes and enzymatic activity). These may result in a change in drug concentration at the site of pharmacologic action with a risk of subsequent toxicity or decreased efficacy respectively. For example, the furanocoumarin extract from grapefruit juice inhibits CYP 450 (3A) which is a key liver isozyme in the metabolism of drugs such as acetaminophen and the antibiotic agent, erythromycin. This inhibitory effect on CYP 450 (3A) will lead to increased plasma concentration of either drug if taken alongside grapefruit juice and may precipitate potential toxic effects. Pharmacodynamic interactions are described by the effects of one drug or medicinal substance being changed by the presence of another drug or substance at its pharmacological site of action. These interactions can be further sub-categorised to additive and synergistic effects or antagonistic (opposing) effects (26). For example, Garlic and Ginger have antiplatelet activity and can increase the risk of bleeding if taken with anticoagulant agents such as Aspirin, a Non-Steroidal Anti-inflammatory Drug (NSAID) and Warfarin.

Some drug interactions are exploited for increased efficacy and reduced toxicity in combination therapy for conditions such as hypertension and other cardiovascular disorders, diabetes mellitus, microbial infections and cancer chemotherapy to name a few. These drug interactions are generally well defined and standardised to produce the desired therapeutic effects. It is likely that medicinal plants that have different phytochemistry will have different pharmacodynamic and pharmacokinetic properties and could be explored for beneficial drug interactions. Likewise, the use of herbal products with characterised and standardised phytochemicals could be used concomitantly with other drugs, once no deleterious drug interactions are anticipated. However, the likelihood exists that medicinal plants with similar taxonomic classification and phytochemistry will have similar pharmacodynamic and pharmacokinetic properties and may lead to toxic effects without careful characterisation and standardisation of the phytoconstituents of either plant. Table 3.2 shows a list of popular sources of drug interactions involving plant-based products and conventional drugs.

The use of herbal remedies is still highly criticised by the medical fraternity due to potential drug-herb interactions as illustrated in table 3.2 and also toxicities associated with some bioactive constituents in

Table 3.2: Popular Drug – Herb Interactions between Medicinal Plants and Conventional Drugs

Ginkgo Biloba	Inhibits platelet aggregation and can interact synergistically with Warfarin & NSAIDS
Garlic	Inhibits platelet aggregation and can interact synergistically with Warfarin & NSAIDS
Ginger	Inhibits platelet aggregation and can interact synergistically with Warfarin & NSAIDS
Turmeric	Inhibits platelet aggregation and can interact synergistically with Warfarin & NSAIDS
Papaya fruit	Inhibits platelet aggregation and can interact synergistically with Warfarin & NSAIDS
Mauby bark	Inhibits platelet aggregation and can interact synergistically with Warfarin & NSAIDS
St John's Wort (hypericum extract)	Increase serotonin levels in the brain significantly when taken with Selective Serotonin Reuptake Inhibitors (SSRIs)
Grapefruit juice (furanocoumarin extract)	Inhibition of CYP 450 (3A) and will increase plasma concentration of acetaminophen, codeine and erythromycin.
Echinacea extracts or products	Reduce hepatic glutathione stores which affect the metabolism of acetaminophen and increase the risk of hepatotoxicity
Aloe vera (emodin)	Increased gastric motility especially with other laxatives. This can affect the rate of absorption of other drugs
Yellow Foxglove (extracts)	Cardiac glycoside effects which can precipitate cardiotoxicity with other cardiac glycosides e.g., Digoxin

NSAIDS – Nonsteroidal anti-inflammatory drugs

plants which remain uncharacterised (56). In order for medicinal plants to be used along with conventional drugs for the same desired outcome, both medicinal products need to be characterised and standardised, and the doses of either or both might need to be adjusted to prevent adverse drug reactions and resulting toxicities.

In summary, drug interactions become more critical when conventional drugs and plant-based remedies or a combination of plant-based preparations are used with an unawareness of the phytochemical profile of the plant-based remedies. The uncharacterised phytochemicals in the plants present the risk of many unknown drug-herb or herb-herb interactions, which can precipitate toxic effects or in some instances, lessen the therapeutic effect of a conventional drug or the more promising medicinal preparation. Moreover, drug interactions from uncharacterised phytochemicals could be potentially beneficial but are problematic for therapeutic monitoring. Some plants may also possess compounds with narrow therapeutic dose ranges that pose serious health effects by virtue of toxicity, especially when administered to vulnerable groups such as infants, persons suffering from liver and kidney disorders and the elderly. In such cases, drug or herbal preparation doses must be closely monitored. The use of extracts from the Yellow Foxglove plant is a key example of a botanical medicine with compounds which may pose risks due to a narrow therapeutic dosing range.

4

Development of Medicinal Plants into Drugs and Medicines

DRUG DEVELOPMENT PIPELINE

Medicinal plants are the precursors to modern medicine and a significant portion of developed drugs are derived from phytochemistry (26, 65). The subdiscipline of pharmacology which focuses on the development of drugs from natural sources is Pharmacognosy, but this area is not only limited to plants but micro-organisms and other biotic sources. Morphine, atropine, cocaine, vincristine, metformin, and digoxin are a few examples of drugs developed from plants and accessed as conventionl medicines. Drugs that are developed go through an extensive series of laboratory, animal, and human studies to determine efficacy and safety. This is called the drug development pipeline. The process is divided into three critical components: drug discovery, preclinical development, and clinical development.

Drug Discovery

Drug discovery involves the selection of candidate molecules based on their pharmacological properties and generally takes 2–5 years in duration. It starts with selecting the specific biological target which is central to the disease to be treated. Receptors, ion channels, enzymes and transporter proteins are the main drug targets; however, there are non-protein targets, such as nucleic acid, ribonucleic acid (RNA) and deoxynucleic acid (DNA) which can be targeted by a wide range of chemotheraputic agents. The next critical step in Drug Discovery is **Lead Finding.** During this step, an assay system is used to determine the functional activity of the biological target. The assays can be enzymatic, membraned-based receptor binding or otherwise, but related to a cellular response. Plant based compounds have been identified as good sources of compounds which can interact with enzymes as inhibitors. Lead finding also involves combinatorial chemistry, which facilitates a large number of related compounds being tested. These compounds could be derived within a given solvent extract from a plant. The development of methods for dereplication, extraction and pre-fractionation of extracts has improved the efficiency of lead finding from plants immensely. Compounds that are successful in interacting with the drug target are maintained for further testing, but some compounds have unfavourable attributes, which may be undesirable in medicines. Some of these attributes are quite prominent among phytochemicals and could include high molecular weights, excessive polarity and possession of chemical groups known to be associated with toxicity (69, 101). Also, the therapeutic properties of plant extracts are sometimes related to the synergistic and simultaneous action of several phytochemicals referred to as "the entourage effect"(102). Table 4.1 highlights some limitations and potential solutions affiliated with the use of natural products for drug discovery (69).

The next critical step in Drug Discovery is **Lead Optimisation** which is increasing the potency of the compounds identified from *lead finding*. Traditionally, this step may include some synthesis (chemical and biosynthesis) to create analogues of compounds with better selectivity to biological targets associated with a disease and improved metabolic stability. However, related compounds in specific plant extracts with better selectivity and metabolic stability can be considered rather than synthetic analogues. Apart from the biological assays described earlier, a broader range of assays can be applied for lead optimisation which may include *in vivo* testing in animals to check for bioactivity, *in vivo* time

Table 4.1. Limitations and Solutions of Bioactivity-Guided Extraction and Isolation of Natural product Compounds for Drug Discovery

Bioactivity-Guided Isolation Steps	Associated Limitations	Solutions
Extraction of compounds from natural sources	Difficulty in producing the organism with consistent chemotypes outside its natural habitat. Relevant phytochemicals may no longer be produced consistently when taken out of the natural habitat.	Propagation and amelioration of plant species with specific attributes and the propagation of specific varieties. Biosynthesis using microorganisms (Fungi) to increase and develop analogues for lead finding and optimisation.
Identification of crude extract with promising pharmacological activity	Presence of compounds that are already known. Presence of compounds that lack drug-like properties. Insufficient amounts of compounds for characterisation.	Development of methods for: dereplication, extraction, and pre-fractionation of extracts.
Isolation of pure bioactive compound through consecutive bioactivity-guided fractionation	Significant time and effort needed to determine the affected molecular targets.	Development of methods for accelerated elucidation of molecular modes of action.

course assays, side effects and oral bioavailability. Upon the completion of these three key steps of Drug Discovery, the successfully extracted single compounds from the plants are considered **drug candidates** and can be introduced to preclinical development (26).

Preclinical Development

The preclinical development of drug candidates ensures that these compounds meet safety requirements before human trials and is usually 1–2 years in duration. In 2008, 46 out of 99 natural products in the global drug development pipeline were identified as being derived from plants(101). Most of these were for use as anti-cancer agents and anti-infectives, and were a fraction of a 30% reduction in overall projects of natural product-based development between 2001 and 2008. These studies occur mainly in animals, and good laboratory practices are generally employed while undergoing these investigations.

Preclinical development comprises of pharmacological testing, preliminary toxicological testing, pharmacokinetic testing, and chemical and pharmacological development. Pharmacological testing focuses on the safety of the drug candidates and identifies any respiratory, cardiovascular and muscular abnormalities related to the administration of the potential drug. Toxicological testing is to identify and eliminate genotoxicity, establishing the therapeutic index (safety dosing range), identifying any cellular, morphological and biochemical abnormalities, and checking for gross changes inclusive of weight-loss. Pharmacokinetic testing is centred on the absorption, distribution, metabolism, and excretion of the drug candidates. Unlike the development of most drugs, plant-based natural product compounds are not amenable to large scale-up due to the complexity of their chemical structure (69). However, biosynthesis can be employed using micro-organisms like bacteria and fungi. The stability of the compounds is also assessed and used to guide formulations for clinical trials. Fifty percent of the drug candidates fail during this stage of development. Successful compounds are well documented and submitted to the relevant regulatory authorities for a Notice of Claimed Investigational Exemption for a New Drug (IND). After this stage, some preclinical work will continue as the drug candidates are tested for long-term toxicity, primarily on fertility and foetal development.

DEVELOPMENT OF MEDICINAL PLANTS INTO DRUGS AND MEDICINES

Clinical Development

Clinical development of drug compounds proceeds through four distinct phases; Phase I, Phase II, Phase III and Phase IV trials/studies and is the longest segment of the drug development pipeline. On average, the first 3 phases can last 6–9 years with no set duration on Phase IV. Phase I trials, which are generally performed on 20–80 normal healthy volunteers, are used to determine safety, tolerability, and pharmacokinetic properties of the **development compound**. In some instances, there are also studies that investigate the mechanism of action of the drug candidates in humans. Phase II trials are generally performed on 100–300 patients and are used for testing the efficacy of the development compound in the clinical situation. It is also used to establish the dosage and sample size for Phase III trials. Phase III trials are usually performed on 1,000–3,000 patients and compare the new drug with other alternatives (i.e. standard therapy or placebo). This stage of drug development is extremely costly and may take a few years especially if the drug is for the treatment of a chronic condition. At the end of Phase III trials, developers of the drugs engage regulatory entities such as the United States Food and Drug Administration (USFDA) and equivalent agencies around the world to submit a New Drug Application/Biologics License Application (NDA/BLA). Approximately two-thirds of submissions gain marketing approval. All the stages of the clinical development require extensive documentation and must follow Good Clinical Practice. The last stage of clinical development is Phase IV trials which involves obligatory post marketing surveillance to determine any rare long-term adverse effects in thousands of patients. It is by this phase that some drugs or batches of production are recalled by the regulatory bodies for further assessment (26).

In 2008, it was reported that 62 plant derived development compounds from 126 natural product compounds were in clinical development (101). Approximately 1 in 50 drug discovery projects will be successful and the development process takes 12 years on average. Phase III trials and long-term toxicity studies (from preclinical studies to clinical development) are the longest and most expensive segments of the drug development pipeline. Moreover, the amount of time required for drug development can be accelerated based on the urgency of the use of the drug under development, for example, vaccines for public health emergencies. During the COVID-19 pandemic, effective and safe vaccines were produced within months rather than years (103). The accelerated time was due to pooled resources for the scientific assessments and the use of drug delivery mechanisms of the vaccines which were previously developed. Further, some vaccines were provided with emergency use approval status and were allowed to be used as a public health strategy against the transmission of the Severe Acute Respiratory Syndrome Coronavirus 2.

CANNABIS: PROHIBITIVE SHIFTS AND THE DEVELOPMENT OF A MEDICINAL CANNABIS INDUSTRY

The Caribbean is recognised as one of the top plant biodiversity hotspots globally. The cultural convergence of ancestral practices has added to this diverse repertoire of traditional knowledge on the use of medicinal plants and biocultural diversity. The plants have been explored multiple times for the development of pharmaceutical products and wellness-based natural products. Some of these examples include Madagascar Periwinkle (*Catharanthus roseus*), Bay Leaf (*Pimenta racemosa*), Ginger (*Zingiber officinale*) and Lemon Grass (*Cymbopogon citratus*). The most compelling example of the exploration of a plant in Barbados and in a few other Caribbean territories for medicinal properties is Medicinal Cannabis. In the next sections of the chapter, Cannabis will be explored as an illustration of a value chain approach and value-added commodity for the scientific development of a medicinal plant for pharmaceutical and wellness industries. Cannabis is controversial due to its controlled status globally and the history of its prohibition.

The Cannabis plant belongs to the plant family Cannabaceae and exists as three sub-species of *Cannabis sativa* inclusive of ssp. sativa, spp. indica and spp. ruderalis. The use of Cannabis dates back to 5000 years on the continents of Asia and Europe (104). Prior to its prohibition, it was extensively used for sociocultural practices; especially as a medicine, and Cannabis extracts were included in the United States Pharmacopeia (USP) until 1940 in USPXII. Prohibition dates to the passing of the Marijuana Tax Act of 1937 in the United States. However, a more thorough review of prohibition against Cannabis identifies the inclusion of 'hashish' or Indian hemp in the list of dangerous substances to be controlled by international legislation following the Hague (1912) and Geneva (1924–25) Opium conventions as the defining moment for Cannabis prohibition. This led to the herb being reclassified in the West Indies under the 1937 Dangerous Drug Ordinance. Prior to this period, Cannabis was commonly consumed, cultivated and a culturally acceptable substance by the East Indian populations in Trinidad and Tobago, Guyana and Jamaica (105). Global prohibitive policies as evidenced in the United Nations Office on Drugs and Crime's Single Convention on Narcotic Drugs 1961 and its Convention on Psychotropic Drugs 1971 which govern the control of narcotic and psychotropic substances have informed legislation and drug policies in signatory countries. Article 4 (c) of the Single Convention on Narcotics 1961 has provisions for countries to lawfully explore the production, manufacture, export, import, distribution, trade and use of Cannabis for its medicinal and scientific purposes. It is under these provisions that Cannabis law reform towards the establishment of Cannabis industries has been the focus. California decriminalised Cannabis in 1996 (106). In 2021, 37 states of the United States of America along with District of Columbia, Guam and Puerto Rico have passed or was in the process of passing Medicinal Cannabis Laws. At that time, Cannabis was is also legal in 17 states and 2 US territories. These policy reforms against prohibition of Cannabis across North America occurred during the transitionary period of Canada's Cannabis regime from a medicinal framework in 2001 towards full legalisation of the use of Cannabis on October 18, 2018. The passing of the Cannabis Act in 2018 made Canada the first G-20 country to legalise recreational Cannabis. At that time, Cannabis was also legal in Uruguay, Georgia, and South Africa but with regulations. Countries in Europe, West Africa, Asia, and Australia have also embraced Medicinal Cannabis.

Prohibitive shifts in the Caribbean Community

In the last decade, the Caribbean Community (CARICOM) has transitioned from its prohibitive policy against Cannabis to a more liberal stance (107, 108). Jamaica was the first of the Caribbean territories to amend its Dangerous Drug Act to decriminalise Cannabis for recreational purposes in 2015. The Jamaica Dangerous Drugs (Amendment) Act established the legal framework to cultivate Cannabis for scientific and medical purposes. More so, to facilitate the activities of a Medicinal Cannabis industry. Section 6(2) of the Act made provision for the lawful prescription of Medicinal Cannabis products by a registered medical practitioner approved by the Ministry of Health and Wellness. In 2018, the CARICOM Regional Commission on Marijuana recommended that Cannabis should be reclassified based on its medicinal benefits and supported the development of a Medicinal Cannabis industry as a potential economic engine for the Caribbean (108). By the close of 2020, other CARICOM member and associate member states inclusive of Antigua and Barbuda, Belize, Dominica, St. Kitts and Nevis and St. Vincent and the Grenadines, Trinidad and Tobago and the US Virgin Island had passed legislation for decriminalisation for the possession of up to a specific quantity of Cannabis ranging from 8–54 grams and cultivation of a limited number (< 6) of plants on private property. By the close of 2020, all these countries have or were in the process of implementing a legislative framework for pursuing Medicinal Cannabis industries to regulate the commercial production and use of Cannabis as a medicine. The Cayman Islands have legislation allowing for the prescribing and use of imported oils and tinctures as medicines. These policy changes were further supported with the reclassification of Cannabis by the United Nations's Commission on Narcotic Drugs by removing Cannabis from schedule 4 of the Single Convention on Narcotics 1961, thus recognising its medicinal value.

Cannabis Reform in Barbados

In 2019, the Government of Barbados implemented a phased approach towards access to Cannabis for medicinal purposes and the establishment of a Medicinal Cannabis industry. The former was done by utilising the provision of section 12 of the Drug Abuse (Prevention and Control) Act; Chapter 131 to add United States Food and Drug Administration (USFDA) or any other drug regulatory body approved Medicinal Cannabis products to the national formulary. The passing of the legislative framework, The Barbados Medicinal Cannabis Act 2019 facilitated phase 2 of the access to Cannabis for medicinal purposes. The Medicinal Cannabis Industry Act 2019 was passed in Parliament and the House of Assembly in the latter part of 2019. The Barbados Medicinal Cannabis Industry Regulations were developed and approved in 2020 and the industry was launched in January 2021. The regime allows the development of a regulated value chain to facilitate the cultivation, manufacturing, research and development, retail and distribution, importation and exportation, testing and consumption of Medicinal Cannabis (107). In 2019, the Government also developed the Sacramental Cannabis Bill which was approved by Parliament and the House of Assembly that would allow Rastafarians to access and use Cannabis at their place of worship. In 2021, the Government advanced its position in the Throne Speech of then Governor General to decriminalise the possession of up to 14 grams of Cannabis and reduce its penalty for possession of such amounts or less to a ticked offence.

Cannabis as a Medicine

The Cannabis plant should be regarded as a catalyst for the exploration of other plants for medicinal and economic benefits. The highly touted medicinal compounds within the Cannabis plant are known as phytocannabinoids. These are secondary metabolites which are synthesized and stored in the trichomes of the plant's inflorescence. Apart from the cannabinoids, there are terpenes, sterols and flavonoids which are also important in producing the health effects of Cannabis (109). There are approximately 125 phytocannabinoids identified in the plant and the most popular bioactive phytocannabinoids are delta-9-tetrahydrocannabinol (THC), cannabidiol (CBD) and cannabinol (CBN). The phytocannabinoids bind primarily to cannabinoid receptors, CB1 and CB2, in the endocannabinoid system (ECS) found in the central nervous system and peripheral sites respectively in all vertebrates. There have also been reports of the interaction of cannabinoids (both endogenous and exogenous) with other types of receptors inclusive of the Glycoprotein Receptor 55 (GPR55), Peroxisome-Proliferator Activated Receptors (PPARs) and the Transient Receptor Potential (TRP) Channels (110, 111). The ECS is activated by the binding of endogenous ligands called endocannabinoids such as anandamide and 2-arachdonoyl-glycerol, the two most characterised endocannabinoids, which are regulated by metabolising enzymes, Monoacylglycerol Lipase and Fatty Acid Amide Hydrolase. It can also be activated by synthetic, and plant derived cannabinoids. The ECS modulates physiological processes including appetite stimulation, analgesia, pleasure sensation, immune response, memory, mood, pre and post-natal development and memory (109, 110). It also facilitates the pharmacological effects of the cannabinoids.

Up to 2019, the USFDA had approved four cannabinoid-formulated products (112). Epidiolex (CBD) has been approved for the treatment of infantile epileptic seizures associated with Lennox-Gastaut syndrome and Dravet syndrome. Marinol and Syndros (Dronabinol [synthetic THC]) in capsule and oral solution formulations respectively, have been approved for therapeutic uses in the United States, including the treatment of anorexia associated with weight loss in acquired immunodeficiency syndrome (AIDS) patients. Cesamet (Nabilone [synthetic THC]) in a capsule formulation has been approved for nausea and emesis associated with cancer chemotherapy (112). There has been modest quality evidence, supporting the use of cannabinoid therapy in chronic, neuropathic and cancer related pain, spasticity related to multiple sclerosis or paraplegia and appetite stimulation in cancer patients (113). In 1987, Professor Manley West, a pharmacologist at the Faculty of Medical Sciences of The University of the West Indies, Mona and Dr. Albert Lockhart, an ophthalmologist, developed Canasol to treat glaucoma and Asthmasol to treat asthma from Cannabis.

SWOT Analysis of Medicinal Cannabis Industry in the Caribbean

The Medicinal Cannabis Industry includes activities and professionals that are involved directly or indirectly in the legal production, transport, sale and consumption or use of Medicinal Cannabis (107). The following represents a Strengths, Weaknesses, Opportunities and Threats (SWOT) analysis of the Medicinal Cannabis industry in the Caribbean:

Strengths

1. Extensive use of the plant to treat ailments dating to 5000 years inclusive of:
    a. Validated scientific approaches for the use of phytoconstituents (109, 114).
    b. Precedent on Medicinal Cannabis regulations established by Canada, the first G-20 nation to legalise Cannabis.
2. The CARICOM Regional Commission on Marijuana recommended that Cannabis should be reclassified based on its medicinal benefits and supported the development of a Medicinal Cannabis industry as a potential economic engine for the Caribbean (108).
3. Niche areas of strength across the value chain with the potential to stimulate economic activity in the Caribbean for example, cultivation, research and development on cultivars, products and clinical applications are present.
4. The legal Cannabis industry was expected to grow towards US$444 billion globally by 2030. The Medicinal Cannabis Industry has been projected to occupy about 33% of that amount (115).

Weaknesses

1. Prohibitive legislation and its impact on research on the medicinal value of Cannabis.
    a. Use of Cannabis is limited for medicinal and scientific purposes

as prescribed by the UN Single Convention for Narcotic Drugs 1961 and UN Convention for Psychotropic Drugs 1971.
2. Social injustices associated with the prosecution of minor offenders during the prohibition phase detracts from Medicinal Cannabis in Caribbean states (107).
3. Cost of procuring a license and a complicated licensure process may be prohibitive to some practitioners and researchers (116).
4. Untrained and uncertified workforce across value chain.
    a. Low uptake of Continual Professional Education (CPE) by healthcare workers.
    b. Technical and vocational training opportunities on Cannabis limited in the Caribbean.
5. Licensees may find it difficult to adjust and adhere to global quality standards inclusive of Good Agricultural and Collection Practices (GACP), Good Manufacturing Practices (GMP), Good Production Practices (GPP) and European Union – Good Manufacturing Practices (EU-GMP).
6. Lack of appropriate equipment for genetic and chemical fingerprinting in the Caribbean.

Opportunities

1. Multiple avenues for the generation of Intellectual Property through research across the value chain.
    a. Extended period of prohibition has created a wealth of research opportunities in pharmacology and clinical applications (113).
    b. Caribbean's geographical location, unique land topography and chemical composition may lead to regionally developed cultivars.
2. The Hemp Farming Act of 2018 removed hemp (defined as Cannabis with less than 0.3% THC) from Schedule I controlled substances in the USA making it an ordinary agricultural commodity.
3. The House of Representatives in the US voted to pass the Secure and Fair Enforcement (SAFE) Banking Act 2019 and 2021 to protect banks that work with the Cannabis industry with the USA.

a. The possibility exists for electronic money systems to safeguard the trade of Cannabis with block chain technology.
4. A potential source for developing alternative energy (biofuel) by the use of the biomass of Cannabis after extraction (117).
5. Stimulate a viable economy from the value chain of Medicinal Cannabis in the Caribbean.
    a. Direct and indirect Cannabis employment opportunities derived from the value chain enterprises.
    b. Cooperatives to assist small and medium size enterprises or businesspeople.
    c. Potential inter-sectorial linkages with Tourism, Agriculture, Education and Health exit.

Threats

1. Acute and chronic adverse effects of delta-9-tetrahydrocannabinal (THC) based formulations and potential drug interactions exist (118, 119).
2. Restricted list of qualifying conditions for the use of Medicinal Cannabis locally and regionally (116).
3. Patents may have been issued to more advanced laboratories and other research-based entities in other jurisdictions which have been researching Cannabis during the prohibition period.
4. US Federal laws still classify Cannabis as a schedule 1 drug which denotes no medicinal value.
5. Banking of Cannabis businesses is problematic in the western hemisphere due to money laundering risk aversion and the need to trade through US corresponding banks which are governed by US federal law.
6. The high cost of Medicinal Cannabis products currently on formulary is prohibitive.
7. Some elements of cultivation & production can be challenging.
    a. Diversion of Cannabis between legal and illegal trades (116).
    b. Maintenance of seed genetics and cultivar chemotypes can be difficult to stabilize.

c. Use of arable land for Cannabis versus crop production is a potential concern for food security.
   d. Cost of indoor and greenhouse cultivation may be prohibitive in the Caribbean setting.
   e. Growth quality issues due to fluctuations in environmental factors.
8. Over regulation of the Medicinal Cannabis industry (116).

CONSIDERATIONS

The traditional use of herbal or botanical medicine in Barbados (and the wider Caribbean) can be viewed as being derived from a rich convergence of biocultural practices. It has survived centuries and is still active in local culture. According to chapter 2 which details traditional and current practices of the plants as medicines, close to 100% of these plant entries identified for the treatment of diseases in Barbados contain pharmacologically active phytochemicals, and a similar amount of the plant entries had studies reporting activities consistent with their reported use.

It is anticipated that such findings on efficacy and safety of plants will continue to support medinical uses of plants as more targeted research is done globally. This work provides a comprehensive guide along with empirical evidence on the phytochemistry and uses of medicinal plants spanning the past two centuries in Barbados. Approved conventional drug compounds or active pharmaceutical ingredients with similar chemical structure to some of these bioactive compounds from the medicinal plants were found to a lesser extent but supports the scientific merit of plants or their extracts as derivatives of medicine. Potential prohibitive factors were identified in the development of natural compounds from plants to pharmaceutical products. This is also compounded with the long turnaround of the drug discovery pipeline and success rate of projects from drug discovery to clinical development. The data entries identify phytochemicals which have proven to be useful in pre-clinical and clinical trials. However, use of plants as medicinal alternatives to conventional medicines without careful guidance must be cautioned until robust efficacy and safety evidence substantiates their uses. The second edition of *Medicinal Plants of Barbados* outlines some important considerations on the use of these remedies especially with concomitant use with conventional drugs. As mentioned previously, polypharmacy is a practice that involves the use of multiple drugs to alleviate an illness, inclusive of the use of plant-based remedies with conventional medicines. In the region, it would be safe to speculate that polypharmacy has a higher frequency than reported in pharmacovigilance programmes because of the lack of trust and rapport between patients and physicians due to fear of being reprimanded for "unconventional" practices. Possible drug-herb interactions can cause additive or synergistic effects leading to toxicity. In some instances, they may lead to the loss of the pharmacological action of the conventional drugs or an increased therapeutic effect. The latter, though a desirable outcome, will need to be clearly researched, documented and standardised to be exploited clinically.

Extensive research on botanical medicines has been done in other Caribbean territories such as Jamaica, Trinidad and Tobago, and Guyana in comparison to Barbados. It is anticipated that this book will increase the volume of work used to assess the potential uses of medicinal plants. The focus of the suggested investigations should be on standardisation of bioactive compounds, therapeutic dosing of these plant compounds, toxicity, and drug-herb interactions. This research could foster the development of natural products from these plant sources and be a possible driver for further economic development of Barbados and the Caribbean. Works produced in this book, TRAMIL and other ethnopharmacology researchers in the Caribbean have established the groundwork for these developments. The explored benefits of these plants could also be used to generate greater awareness and use of the plants in their raw form using safe practices. These prospects should be geared toward the blooming health and wellness sector, which is associated with the preventative, therapeutic and rehabilitative care provided to ailing and non-ailing individuals. This sector is a prime candidate to mobilize regional development given the potential use of natural products from the region as a unique selling point. The medicinal Cannabis industry in Barbados and in the Caribbean is a key example of the exploration of medicinal plants as a potential economic driver. However, there are at least 157 entries of medicinal plant uses in Barbados that are less prohibitive than controlled narcotic plants. These opportunities to produce innovative, value-added products will establish the Caribbean as a recognizable brand globally. Possible product categories are fortified/functional foods, nutraceuticals, pharmaceuticals and cosmeceuticals. It is anticipated that the region's rich plant and food diversity, and the research and development of medicinal plants will boost the development of health and wellness products, the health of the people through socially inclusive practices and build regional economies.

Glossary of Terms

WORD	DEFINITION
Active pharmaceutical ingredient	This is the biologically active component of a drug that produces the intended effects
Antineoplastic agents	These are drugs which inhibit or prevent the development of neoplasia.
Bioactive	Of or relating to a substance that has an effect on living tissue.
Biocultural	A combination of biological and cultural factors that affect human behaviour
Botanical	Of or relating to plants or plant life.
Communicable disease	These are also known as transmissible diseases and comprise clinically evident illness, resulting from an infection, presence and growth of pathogenic biological agents in an individual host organism.
Conventional	Based on or in accordance with general agreement, use, or practice.
Decoction	To make concentrated or to boil for varied lengths of time
Drug	Administered substance of known structure(s), other than a nutrient or an essential dietary ingredient, which, when administered produces an effect on biological systems.
Drug-herb interaction	The direct and indirect interaction between a drug and herbal substance in the body from concurrent use of both substances. The interaction may lead to mimicking, magnification, or an opposition of the effects of either substance.

GLOSSARY OF TERMS

WORD	DEFINITION
Efficacy	The capacity to produce an effect. More specifically in medicine, the capacity to produce a beneficial or therapeutic effect.
Endemic	Belonging or native to a particular people or country and found nowhere else
Ethnopharmacology	The scientific study of materials used by ethnic and cultural groups as medicines
Folklore	The traditional beliefs, customs, and stories of a community, passed through generations by word of mouth.
Herb	Any plant used for flavouring, food, medicine, or perfume.
Herbal substance	a preparation of a plant or an extract or a mixture of these
Herb-herb interaction	The direct and indirect interaction between two herbal substances in the body from concurrent use of both substances. The interaction may lead to mimicking, magnification, or an opposition of the effects of either substance.
Horticulturist	An expert in the science of cultivating plants (fruit, flowers, vegetables or ornamental plants).
Indication *(medicine)*	Something that points to or suggests the proper treatment of a disease, as that demanded by its cause or symptoms.
Indigenous	Originating in and characteristic of a particular region or country.
Infusion	A drink or extract prepared by soaking part(s) of a plant (e.g., leaves, stem or roots) in liquid and can be hot or cold
Neoplasm	An abnormal growth of body tissue. It can be cancerous (malignant) or noncancerous (benign).

GLOSSARY OF TERMS

WORD	DEFINITION
Non-communicable disease (NCD)	A medical condition or disease which is non-infectious and non-transmissible between persons.
Nutraceutical	Foodstuff (as a fortified food or a dietary supplement) that provides health or medical benefits in addition to its basic nutritional value.
Pharmaceutical	Relating to or engaged in the manufacture and sale of drugs.
Pharmacognosy	The study of drugs of natural origins or sources.
Pharmacokinetic antagonism	The use of a drug or substance which affects the concentration of the active drug or substance at the pharmacological site of action.
Pharmacology	The study of the effects of chemical substances on the functions of living systems.
Phylogeny	The evolutionary development and history of a species.
Phytochemical	Chemical constituents of plants with discrete bioactivities towards animal biochemistry and metabolism.
Polypharmacy	A practice that involves the use of multiple drugs to alleviate an illness especially when all the treatment forms are not clinically warranted.
Poultice	A soft and moist mass of material, typically of plant material or flour, applied to the body to relieve soreness and inflammation and can be kept in place with a cloth.
Primary	First or highest in rank, quality, or importance; principal.
Secondary	Second in rank, quality, or importance.

WORD	DEFINITION
Steeping	The soaking of organic matter for example tea, in water or other liquid to extract its flavour.
Synergism *(medicine - drugs)*	The additive effect of two drugs to produce an effect greater than the sum of their individual effects.
Systematic review	A literature review that tries to identify, appraise, select, and synthesize all high-quality research evidence addressing a research question.
Tertiary	Third in rank, quality, or importance.

Bibliography

1. Poyer J. The history of Barbados, from the first discovery of the island in the year 1605 till the accession of Lord Seaforth, 1801. London: J G Barnard, Printer, Snow Hill; 1808.
2. Lane A. Race, Class, and Development in Barbados Caribb. Q. 1979;25(1/2):40–51.
3. CARICOM. The West Indian Federation: CARICOM; 2021 [updated 31/03/2021]. Available from: https://caricom.org/the-west-indies-federation/.
4. Phillips ADV, Marshall WK, Jackson CS. Barbados Encylcopaedia Britanica; 2025. Available from: https://www.britannica.com/place/Barbados/Climate.
5. CARICOM. The Caribbean Commity: Who we are: CARICOM; 2021 [updated 31/03/2021; cited CARICOM 03/04/2021]. Available from: https://caricom.org/our-community/who-we-are/.
6. Barbados Statistical Service. Visitor Arrivals – December 2024 Statistical Bulletin. Bridgetown, Barbados: Barbados Statistical Service; 2024.
7. Barbados Integrated Government. Demographics. 2021. [updated 2021. Available from: https://www.gov.bb/Visit-Barbados/demographics.
8. United Nations Devlopment Programme. Human Development Reports. United Nations Development Programme; 2020 [cited 2021]. http://hdr.undp.org/en/countries/profiles/BRB#.
9. World Health Organisation. Global health observatory data repository Geneva: World Health Organisation; 2021 [updated 07/05/2018]. Available from: http://apps.who.int/gho/data/view.main
10. Moonie S, Quashie N. Social health protection for the elderly in the English-speaking Caribbean. Port of Spain: ECLAC, United Nations; 2011.
11. Handler JS. Diseases and medical disabilities of enslaved Barbadians, from the seventeenth century to around 1838: Part 1. J Caribb. Hist. 2006;40:1–38.
12. Quach H, Rotival M, Pothlichet J, Loh Y-HE, Dannemann M, Zidane

N, et al. Genetic adaptation and Neandertal admixture shaped the immune system of human populations. Cell. 2016;20(3):643–56.
13. Ruwende C, Hill A. Glucose-6-phosphate dehydrogenase deficiency and malaria. J Mol Med. 1998;76:581–8.
14. Cooper R, Rotini C, Ataman S, Mcgee D, Osatimehin B, Kadiri S, et al. The prevalence of hypertension in seven populations of West African origin. Am J Public Health. 1997;87:160–8.
15. Unwin N, Rose A, George K, Hambleton I, Howitt C. The Barbados Health of the Nation Survey: Core Findings. Chronic Disease Research Centre, The University of the West Indies and the Barbados Ministry of Health. St. Michael, Barbados; 2015.
16. Global Burden of Disease Collaborative Network. Global Burden of Disease Study 2019 (GBD 2019). Seattle: United States of America Institute for Health Metrics and Evaluation; 2020.
17. Pan American Health Organisation. PAHO calls for countries in Latin America and the Caribbean to prepare for possible outbreaks of dengue: Pan American Health Organisation; 2019. Available from: https://www.paho.org/hq/index.php?option=com_content&view=article&id=14994:paho-calls-for-countries-in-latin-america-and-the-caribbean-to-prepare-for-possible-outbreaks-of-dengue&Itemid=1926&lang=en.
18. Escobedo A. SARS-CoV-2/COVID-19: Evolution in the Caribbean islands. Travel Medicine and Infectious Disease. 2020;37.
19. Ramírez-Soto MC, Ortega-Cáceres G, Arroyo-Hernández H. Sex differences in COVID-19 fatality rate and risk of death: An analysis in 73 countries, 2020-2021. Infez Med. 2021;29(3):402–7.
20. Heywood V, Brummitt R, Culham A, Seberg O. Flowering Plant Families of the World. Ontario: Firefly Books; 2007
21. International Botanical Congress. International code of nomenclature for algae, fungi, and plants: International Botanical Congress (IBC); 2017 [Available from: https://www.iapt-taxon.org/nomen/main.php.
22. Carrington SM. Wild Plants of Barbados. 2nd ed. Oxford: MacMillan Publishers; 2007.
23. Bayley I. The bush-teas of Barbados. Journal of Barbados Museum and Historical Society. 1949;16:103–12.
24. TRAMIL. Program of Applied Research to Popular Medicine in the

Caribbean 2017 [updated 2017]. Available from: http://www.tramil.net/en.
25. Ayensu E. Medicinal Plants of the West Indies. Michigan, USA: Reference Publications, Inc.; 1981.
26. Ritter JM, Flower R, Henderson G, Loke YK, MacEwan D, Rang HP. Rang and Dale's Pharmacology. 9th ed. London: Elsevier Limited; 2020.
27. Petrovaska B. Historical review of medicinal plants' usage. Pharmacogn Rev. 2012;6 (11):1–5.
28. Sutherland P, Moodley R, Chevannes B. Caribbean healing traditions: implications for health and mental health. 2nd ed. New York: Routledge; 2014.
29. Nestler G. Traditional Chinese medicine. North American Clinical Medicine. 2002;86(1):63–73.
30. Jaiswal Y, Williams L. A glimpse of Ayurveda – The forgotten history and principles of Indian traditional medicine. J Tradit Complemen Med. 2017;7(1):50–3.
31. Hassi A, Storti G. Globalization and culture: the three H scenarios. Rijecka, Croatia: InTech; 2012 28/02/2021.
32. Glazier S. Aboriginal Trinidad and the Guianas: an historical reconstruction. Journal of the Walter Roth Museum of Anthropology. 1980;3(1):119–24.
33. Berry M. Exploring the potential contributions of Amerindians to West Indian Folk Medicine. Southeastern Geographer. 2005;45(2):239–50.
34. White P. The concept of diseases and health care in African traditional religion in Ghana. HTS Theological Studies. 2015;71(3):1–7.
35. Cook H, Walker T. Circulation of medicine in the early modern Atlantic world. Social History of Medicine 2013;26(3):337–51.
36. Abrahams R. The shaping of folklore traditions in the British West Indies. J Interam Stud. & Wld. Aff. 1967;9(3):456–80.
37. Handler J, Bilby K. Obeah: Healing and protection in West Indian slave life. J Caribb Hist. 2004;38(2):153–83.
38. Proctor R. Early developments in Barbadian education. J Negro Educ. 1980;49(2):184–95.
39. Hander J, Jacoby J. Slave medicine and plant use in Barbados. J Barbados Mus Hist Soc. 1993;41:76–98.

40. Cohall D, Scantlebury-Manning T, Cadogan-McClean C, Lallement A, O'Conner S. The impact of the healthcare system in Barbados (provision of health insurance and the benefit service scheme) on the use of herbal remedies by Christian churchgoers. West Indian Med. J. 2011;60:296–301.
41. Peter S. Medicinal and cooling teas of Barbados. in: African Ethnobotany in the Americas. Voeks R, Rashford J, editors. New York: Springer; 2012.
42. Vujicic T, Cohall D. Knowledge, attitudes and practices on the use of botanical medicines in a rural Caribbean territory. Front Pharmacol. 2021;12:713855.
43. Picking D, Younger N, Mitchell S, Delgoda R. The prevalence of herbal medicine home use and concomitant use with pharmaceutical medicines in Jamaica. J Ethnopharmacol. 2011;137(1):305–11.
44. Clement YN, Morton-Gittens J, Basdeo L, Blades A, Francis M-J, Gomes N, et al. Perceived efficacy of herbal remedies by users accessing primary healthcare in Trinidad. BMC Complement Altern Med. 2007;7(1):4.
45. Ekor M. The growing use of herbal medicines: issues relating to adverse reactions and challenges in monitoring safety. Front. Pharmacol. 2014;4:177.
46. Robinson M, Zhang X. The world medicines situation 2011: traditional medicines: global situation, issues and challenges. Geneva: World Health Organisation; 2011.
47. Adeniyi O, Washington L, Glenn CJ, Franklin SG, Scott A, Aung M, et al. (2021) The use of complementary and alternative medicine among hypertensive and type 2 diabetic patients in Western Jamaica: A mixed methods study. PloS ONE 16(2): e0245163. https://doi.org/10.1371/journal.pone.0245163.
48. Mahibir D, Gulliford M. Use of medicinal plants for diabetes in Trinidad and Tobago. Rev Pan Am Salud Publica (RPSP/PAJPH). 1997;1(3):174–9.
49. Merrit-Charles L. The prevalence of herbal medicine use among surgical patients in Trinidad. Focus Altern Complement Ther. 2011;16(4):266–70.
50. Clement Y, Williams A, Aranda D, Chase R, Watson N, Mohammed R. Medicinal herb use among asthmatic patients attending a specialty

care facility in Trinidad. BMC Complement Altern Med. 2005; 15: 5(3).
51. Luciano-Montalvo C, Boulogne I, Gavillan-Suarez J. A screening for antimicrobial activities of Caribbean herbal remedies. BMC Complement Altern Med. 2013;13:126.
52. Hennis A, Hambleton I, Crichlow S, Fraser H. Health,welfare and aging in Bridgetown, Barbados. SABE 2000. Washington, D.C.; 2005.
53. Barbados Drug Service. Welcome to the Brug Service: Barbados Drug Service; 2017 [updated 27/03/2021. Available from: https://www.gov.bb/Departments/drug-service.
54. Ministry of Health and Wellness Research and Planning Unit. Barbados Health Report 2023. Bridgetown, Barbados; 2024.
55. Pan American Health Organization. Health Systems Profile: Barbados – monitoring and analysing health systems change/reform. Washington, D.C.; 2008.
56. Howell L, Kocbbar K, Saywell R, Zollinger T, Koehler J, Mandzuk C, et al. Use of herbal remedies by Hispanic patients: Do they inform their physician? J Am Board Fam Med. 2006;19:566–78.
57. Gardener J, Grant D, Hutchinson S, Wilks R. The use of herbal teas and remedies in Jamaica. West Indian Med J. 2000;49(4):331–5.
58. Adams O, Carter A. Knowledge, attitudes, practices, and barriers reported by patients receiving diabetes and hypertension primary health care in Barbados: a focus group study. BMC Family Practice. 2011; 12(135).
59. Whitemarsh I. Biomedical ambivalence: Asthma diagnosis, the pharmaceutical, and other contradictions in Barbados. Am Ethnol. 2008;35(1):49–63.
60. Elias M. Cultures of the World: Barbados New York: Times Editions Pte Ltd; 2000.
61. Gohar A, Cashman A, Ward F. Managing food and water security in Small Island States: New evidence from economic modelling of climate stressed groundwater resources. J Hydrol. 2018;569.
62. Turland N, Wiersema J, Barrie F, Greuter W, Hawksworth D, Herendeen P, et al. International Code of Nomenclature for algae, fungi, and plants (Shenzhen Code) adopted by the Nineteenth International Botanical Congress Shenzhen, China, July 2017. Glashütten: Koeltz Botanical Books; 2018. Available from: https://doi.org/10.12705/Code.2018.

63. Hawksworth D. Terms used in bionomenclature: The naming of organisms (and plant communities). Copenhagen: Global Biodiversity Information Facility; 2010.
64. Dillard CJ, German JB. Phytochemicals: nutraceuticals and human health. J Sci Food Agric. 2000;80:1744–56.
65. Springob K, Kutchan TM. Introduction to the different classes of natural products in: Plant-derived natural products: synthesis, function, and application. Osbourn AE, Lanzotti V, editors. New York: Springer Science; 2009.
66. Kumar S, Sumner BW, Sumner LW. Modern plant metabolomics for the discovery and characterization of natural products and their biosynthetic genes in: Comprehensive natural products III. Liu H-WB, Begley TP, editors. Amsterdam: Elsevier; 2020.
67. Agar OT, Tatli, I. Analysis of phenylethanoids and their glycosidic derivatives. in: Recent advances in natural products analysis. Silva AS, Nabavi SF, Saeedi M, Nabavi SM, editors. Amsterdam: Elsevier; 2020.
68. Korman TP, Ames B, Tsai S-CS. Structural enzymology of polyketide synthase: The structure–sequence–function correlation. in Comprehensive Natural Products II. Liu H-WB, Mander L, editors. Amsterdam: Elsevier; 2010.
69. Atanasov A, Zotchev S, Dirsch V, Supuran C, Orhan I, Banach M. Natural products in drug discovery: advances and opportunities. Nat Rev Drug Discov. 2021;20(3):200–16.
70. Havsteen BH. The biochemistry and medical significance of the flavonoids. Pharmacol Ther. 2002;96(2-3):67–202.
71. Khan M, Kihara M, Omoloso A. Anti-microbial activity of Bidens pilosa, Bischofia javanica, Elmerillia papuana and Sigesbekia orientalis. Fitoterapia. 2001;72(6):662–5.
72. Goel G, Makkar H, Francis G, Becker K. Phorbol esters: structure, biological activity, and toxicity in animals. Int J Toxicol. 2007;26:279–88.
73. Igbinosa OO, Igbinosa EO, Aiyegoro OA. Antimicrobial activity and phytochemical screening of stem bark extracts from Jatropha curcas (Linn). African J Pharm Pharmacol. 2009;3:58–62.
74. Dargan D, Subak-Sharpe J. The effect of triterpenoid compounds on uninfected and herpes simplex virus-infected cells in culture. II.

DNA and protein synthesis, polypeptide processing and transport. J Gen Virol. 1986;67:1831–50.

75. Ott M, Thyagarajan S, Gupta S. Phyllanthus amarus suppresses hepatitis B virus by interrupting interactions between HBV enhancer I and cellular transcription factors. Eur J Clin Invest. 1997;27:908–15.

76. Saetae D, Suntornsuk W. Antifungal activities of ethanolic extract from Jatropha curcas seed cake. J Microbiol Biotechnol. 2010;20:319–24.

77. Hubbell S, Wiemer D, Adejare A. An antifungal terpenoid defends a neotropical tree against attack by fungus-growing ants. Oecologia. 1983;60:321–7.

78. Mazroatul C, Deni G, Habibi N, Saputri G. Anti-hypercholesterolemia activity of ethanol extract Peperomia pellucida. Alchemy. 2016;12(1):88–94.

79. Mun'Im A, Ramadhani F, K Chaerani, Amelia L, Arrahman A. Effects of gamma irradiation on microbiological, phytochemical content, antioxidant activity and inhibition of angiotensin converting enzyme (ACE) activity of Peperomia pellucida (L.) Kunth. J Young Pharm. 2017;9(1).

80. Kurniawan A, Saputri F, Rissyelly AI, Mun'lm A. Isolation of angiotensin converting enzyme (ACE) inhibitory activity quercetin from Peperomia pellucida. Int J Pharmtech Res. 2016;9(7):115–21.

81. Nwokocha C. Possible mechanism of action of the hypotensive effect of Peperomia pellucida and interactions between human cytochrome P450 enzymes. Med Aromat Plants. 2012;1(4).

82. Taher M-H, Dawood D, Sanad M, Hassan R. Searching for anti-hyperglycemic phytomolecules of Tecoma stans. Eur J Chem. 2016;7(4):397–404.

83. Wang L, Waltenberger B, Pferschy-Wenzig E, Blunder M, Liu X, Malainer C, et al. Natural product agonists of peroxisome proliferator-activated receptor gamma (PPARγ): a review. Biochemi Pharmacol. 2014;92(1):73–89.

84. Bharti S, Krishnan S, Kumar A, Kumar A. Antidiabetic phytoconstituents and their mode of action on metabolic pathways. Ther Adv Endocrinol Metab. 2018;9(3):81–100.

85. Okoli C, Obidike I, Ezike A, Akah P, Salawu O. Studies on the possible mechanisms of antidiabetic activity of extract of aerial parts of Phyllanthus niruri. Pharm Biol. 2011;49(3):248–55.

86. Amin Z, Alshawsh M, Kassim M, Ali H, Abdulla M. Gene expression profiling reveals underlying molecular mechanism of hepatoprotective effect of Phyllanthus niruri on thioacetamide-induced hepatotoxicity in Sprague Dawley rats. BMC Complement Alternat Med. 2013;13:160.
87. Lee S, Jaganath I, Wang S, Sekaran S. Antimetastatic effects of Phyllanthus on human lung (A549) and breast (MCF-7) cancer cell lines. PLoS One. 2011;6(6):e20994.
88. Pappachen L, Chacko A. Preliminary phytochemical screening and in-vitro cytotoxicity activity of Peperomia pellucida Linn. Pharmacie Globale. 2013;4(8):1-4.
89. Xu S, Li N, Ning M, Zhou C, Yang Q, Wang M. Bioactive compounds from Peperomia pellucida. J Nat Prod. 2006;69(2):247–50.
90. Hseu Y, Wu C, Chang H, Kumar K, Lin M, Che C, et al. Inhibitory effects of Physalis angulata on tumor metastasis and angiogenesis. J Ethnopharmacol. 2011;135(3):762–71.
91. Gao C, Ma T, Luo J, Kong L. Three new cytotoxic withanolides from the Chinese folk medicine Physalis angulata. Nat Prod Commun. 2015;10(12):2059–62.
92. Gao C, Li R, Zhou M, Yang Y, Kong L, Luo J. Cytotoxic withanolides from Physalis angulata. Nat Prod Res. 2018;32(6):676-81.
93. Adjibode A, Tougan P, Youssao A, Mensah G, Hanzen C, Koutinhouin G. Synedrella nodiflora (L.) Gaertn: a review on its phytochemical screening and uses in animal husbandry and medicine. Int J Sci Technol Res. 2015;5(3):436–43.
94. Curry E, Murry D, Yoder C, Fife K, Armstrong V, Nakshatri H, et al. Phase I dose escalation trial of feverfew with standardized doses of parthenolide in patients with cancer. Invest New Drugs. 2004;22:299–305.
95. Lowe H, Steele B, Fouad E, Toyang N, Ngwa N. Antiviral activity of Jamaican medicinal plants and isolated bioactive compounds. Molecules. 2021;26(3):607.
96. Gorg V, Dhar V, Sharma A, Dutt R. Facts about standardisation of herbal medicine: a review. Chin J Integr Med. 2012;10(10):1077–83.
97. Muller PY, Milton MN. The determination and interpretation of the therapeutic index in drug development. Nat Rev Drug Discov. 2012;11.
98. Guengerich FP. Mechanisms of Drug toxicity and relevance

to pharmaceutical development. Drug Metab Pharmacokinet. 2011;26:3–14.
99. Raskin I, Ribnicky D, Komarnytsky S, Ilic N, Poauley A, Borisjuk N et al. Plants and human health in the twenty-first century. Trends Biotechnol. 2002;20:522–31.
100. Delgoda R, Ellington C, Barrett S, Gordon N, Clarke N, Younger N. The practice of polypharmacy involving herbal and prescription medicines in the treatment of diabetes mellitus, hypertension and gastrointestinal disorders in Jamaica. West Indian Med. J. 2004;53(6):400–5.
101. Harvey AL. Natural products in drugs discovery. Drug Discov Today. 2008;13(19/20):894–901.
102. Thomford NE, Senthebane DA, Rowe A, Munro D, Seele P, Maroyi A, et al. Natural products for drug discovery in the 21st century: Innovations for novel drug discovery. Int J Mol Sci. 2018;19:1578.
103. Krammer F. SARS-CoV-2 vaccines in development. Nature. 2020;586(7830):516–27.
104. Nutt D. Drugs Without the Hot Air: Minimising the harms of legal and illegal drugs. Cambridge: UIT Cambridge, 2012.
105. Klein A. Between the death penalty and decriminalization: new directions for drug control in the Commonwealth Caribbean. New W Indian Gu. 2001;75:193–227.
106. Pacula R, Powell D, Heaton P, Sevigny E. Assessing the effects of medical marijuana laws on marijuana use: The devil is in the details. J Policy Anal Manage. 2015;34(1):7–31.
107. Griffith A, Cohall D. Conceptualising a policy framework for the implementation of medical marijuana in the Caribbean territory of Barbados. Drug Sci, Policy Law. 2018;4:1–8.
108. Antoine RMB, Abel W, Best E, Francis FL, Griffith ADD, Gossell-Williams M, et al. Report to the Caribbean community heads of government by the CARICOM regional commission on Marijuana: Waiting to exhale, safeguarding our future through responsible socio-legal policy on Marijuana. Turkeyen, Guyana; 2018.
109. Mechoulam R. The pharmacohistory of Cannabis sativa. in: Cannabinoids as therapeutic agents, Boca Raton. Mechoulam R, editor. Boca Raton. Florida: CRC Press; 1986, 1–19.
110. Pacher P, Batkal S, Kunos G. The endocannabinoid system

as an emerging target of pharmacotherapy. Pharmacol. Rev. 2006;58(3):389–462.
111. Lauckner JE, Jenson JB, Chen H-Y, Lu H-C, Hille B, Mackie K. GPR55 is a cannabinoid receptor that increases intracellular calcium and inhibits M current. Proc Natl Acad Sci U S A. . 2008;105(7):2699–704.
112. United States Food and Drug and Administration. FDA regulation of Cannabis and Cannabis-derived products, including Cannabidiol (CBD): USFDA; 2018 [Available from: https://www.fda.gov/newsevents/publichealthfocus/ucm421168.htm#notapproved.]
113. Whiting PF, Wolff RF, Deshpande S, Nislo MD, Duffy S, Hernnadez A, et al. Cannabinoids for medical use: A systematic review and meta-analysis. J Am Med Assoc. 2015;313(24):2456–73.
114. National Academies of Sciences, Engineering, and Medicine. The health effects of Cannabis and Cannabinoids: The current state of evidence and recommendations for research. Washington, D.C.; 2017.
115. Fortune Business Insights. Cannabis Market Size, Share & COVID-19 Impact Analysis, By Type (Flowers/Buds and Concentrates), By Application (Medical, Recreational (Edibles and Topicals), and Industrial Hemp) By Component (THC-Dominant, Balanced THC & CBD, and CBD Dominant), and Regional Forecast, 2023-2030: Fortune Business Insights; 2025. [Available from: https://www.fortunebusinessinsights.com/industry-reports/cannabis-marijuana-market-100219]
116. Jones S, Porter R, Bishop C. The implementation of medicinal ganja in Jamaica. Int J Drug Policy. 2017;42:115–7.
117. Abraham R, Wong C, Puri M. Enrichment of cellulosic waste Hemp (Cannabis sativa) hurd into non-toxic Microfibres. Materials (Basel). 2016;9(7).
118. Cohen K, Weinstein A. Synthetic and Nnon-synthetic Cannabinoid Drugs and Their Adverse Effects – A review from public health prospective. Front Public Health. 2018;6.
119. Watanabe K, Yamaori S, Funahashi T, Kimura T, Yamamoto I. Cytochrome P450 enzymes involved in the metabolism of tetrahydrocannabinols and cannabinol by human hepatic microsomes. Life Sci. 2007;80(15):1415–9.

Index

Figures are indicated by *f* following the page number.

Achyranthes aspera, 69–70, 69*f*
Aegiphila martinicencis, 48, 48*f*
Africa, 5, 7, 11–12, 14, 149
African diaspora, 5, 7, 11–12, 14–16, 18, 127
African Ethnobotany in the Americas (Voeks and Rashford), 16
Afro-Barbadians, 3, 15–16, 18, 20–21
Afro-Caribbean people, 15, 127
Afrocentricity, 17, 21
Ageratum conyzoides, 52, 52*f*, 70, 70*f*
algae, 126
alkaloids, 10, 128, 129*f*3.1, 133–35
  plant sources of, 26–27, 30–31, 33–34, 36, 39–40, 44–46, 48–49, 51–52, 54, 56–58, 61, 64, 70, 72, 74, 76–78, 80, 82–84, 88, 96
Allium sativum, 13, 50–51, 50*f*, 94, 94*f*, 127, 140–41
Almond, Barbados/Seaside, 38–39, 39*f*
Aloe vera, 30, 52, 63, 70, 89, 96, 141
  photographs of, 30*f*, 52*f*, 63*f*, 70*f*, 89*f*, 96*f*
Amaranthus dubius, 50, 50*f*
Amaryllis, 51, 51*f*

Ambrosia hispida, 37, 37*f*, 71, 71*f*
Amerindians, 1, 5, 11–12, 14, 127
Anglicanism, 3, 15–16, 21
animal testing, 24–26, 29–43, 45, 47–49, 55, 89, 91–92, 94, 98–99, 133–34, 143–44
animals, 10, 22, 24, 128, 132, 138, 143–44, 146, 161
Annona muricata, 26, 31, 35–36, 89, 94–95, 130
  photographs of, 26*f*, 36*f*, 89*f*, 95*f*
Anodyne, 41–42, 42*f*, 80, 80*f*
Anthraquinones, 52, 63, 68, 70, 78, 88
antibacterial medicines, 7, 50–69, 96, 128, 131–32, 140
Antigua and Barbuda, 150
antioxidants, 128, 130
  plant sources of, 26, 30–31, 33, 35, 37, 39–40, 42, 46–47, 49, 51, 53, 72, 74, 78, 93–94, 96–98, 133
ants, 132
Arawak people, 11–12
Arrow Leaf, 80, 80*f*
Arrowroot, 12
Asclepias curassavica, 85–86, 86*f*
Asia, 148–49
Asians, in the Caribbean, 3, 12
asthma, 7, 19, 97, 152

173

INDEX

Australia, 149
Ayensu, Edward S., 9
Ayurveda (traditional Indian medicine), 11, 13–14
Azadirachta indica, 33, 42, 59, 64–65, 90, 98
   photographs of, 33*f*, 42*f*, 59*f*, 65*f*, 90*f*, 98*f*

bacteria, 5, 24, 50–69, 96, 126, 132, 146
Baháʼí Faith, 4, 22
Ball Bush, 78–79, 79*f*
Balsam
   Garden, 34, 35*f*
   Yellow, 76, 76*f*
Barbados
   demographics of, 3–5, 7
   health in, 4–8, 17–20, 131, 138–39
   history of, 1, 3, 14–16, 20
   laws of, 150–51
   map of, 2*f*1.1
   medicinal plants in, 1, 16–20, 22–24, 130–31, 136, 138–39, 156–58
   plants of, 9, 15, 22, 127
   religion in, 20–22
Bay Leaf, 44, 59–60, 65–66, 91, 99, 130, 148
   photographs of, 44*f*, 59*f*, 66*f*, 91*f*, 99*f*
Bayley, Iris, 17
bearded fig-tree, 1
Belize, 150
Benefit Service Scheme, 19
Bible, 21–22

Bidens alba, 71, 71*f*
Bidens pilosa, 30–31, 37, 52–53, 71, 127, 132
   photographs of, 31*f*, 37*f*, 53*f*
Bilberry, 56–57, 57*f*
bioactive compounds, 24, 130, 135, 145, 156–57
   plant sources of, 46, 48, 72, 88
birds, 138
Bloodroot, 35, 35*f*, 94, 94*f*
Bontia daphnoides, 43–44, 44*f*
Borrichia arborescens, 72, 72*f*
botanical families, 135. *See also* taxonomy
Britain, 1, 3
British empire, 1, 3, 18
Broomweed, 42, 42*f*
Buttonweed, 46, 46*f*, 82–83, 82*f*, 83*f*

Caesarweed, 81, 81*f*
California, 149
Calotropis procera, 29, 29*f*, 86, 86*f*
Canada, 149, 153
cancer, 5, 7–8, 19, 24, 128, 140, 146, 160
   medicinal plants for, 26–28, 95, 97–98, 134–35, 152
Cannabis sativa, 22, 148–49, 155–58
   legality of, 149–51, 153–56
   medicinal uses of, 151–52
Capraria biflora, 61–62, 62*f*, 83, 83*f*
Capsicum annuum, 68, 68*f*, 92, 92*f*
cardiovascular disease, 5–7, 24, 29–30, 133, 140, 146
Carib people, 11–12

INDEX

Caribbean Community (CARICOM), 3, 150, 153n.2
Caribbean Free Trade Association (CARIFTA), 3
Caribbean region, 1, 3, 11–12, 21, 150, 153–58
 health in, 5, 7–8, 131
 medicinal plants in, 9, 11, 13–15, 18, 20, 127, 135, 138–39, 148
Carica papaya, 27, 38, 55, 75, 90, 141
 photographs of, 27*f*, 55*f*, 75*f*, 90*f*
Carpet Daisy, 53, 53*f*
Castor Oil, 58–59, 58*f*, 61
Catharanthus roseus, 27, 27*f*, 36, 36*f*, 134–35, 148
Catholicism, 3–4, 20–21
Cayman Islands, 150
Cecropia schreberiana, 32, 32*f*, 38, 38*f*
Cedar, 21–22
Cerasee, 32, 39, 76, 96–97, 130
 photographs of, 32*f*, 39*f*, 76*f*, 97*f*
Chamaesyce hirta, 57–58, 58*f*, 87, 87*f*
Chicago, 7
chicken pox, 6, 24
Chigger Nut, 55, 55*f*
China, 13
 traditional medicine of, 10, 13, 15
Chiococca alba, 60, 60*f*
Christianity, 3–4, 15–16, 18, 20–22
Christmas Candle, 88, 88*f*
Christmas Hope, 31, 31*f*, 133

chronic conditions, 5–9, 16, 23, 131, 139, 147, 152, 155
Chronic Non-communicable Disease Registry, 7
Citrus limon, 34, 34*f*
cloves, 14
Coconut, 96, 96*f*
Cocos nucifera, 96, 96*f*
Cohall, Damian H., 16
colonialism, 1, 3, 12, 18–22
common cold, 6, 24, 70–74, 76–83, 86
common names, multiple, 127
communicable diseases, 5, 50-88, 130–32, 135, 159
Conga Lala, 72, 72*f*
Congo jute, 81, 81*f*
Cooper, R., 7
COVID-19, 4, 8, 148
Cow Pops, 28–29, 29*f*, 47, 47*f*, 134
Crapaud, 32, 39, 76, 96–97,130
 photographs of, 32*f*, 39*f*, 76*f*, 97*f*
Croton flavens, 76, 76*f*
Croton lechleri, 76
Cucumber, 56, 56*f*
Cucumis sativus, 56, 56*f*
Curcuma longa, 49, 62–63, 68–69, 92–93, 100, 141
 photographs of, 49*f*, 63*f*, 68*f*, 93*f*, 100*f*
Cure-for-All, 73, 74*f*, 132
Cymbopogon citratus, 66–67, 81, 91, 99, 127, 148
 photographs of, 67*f*, 81*f*, 91*f*, 99*f*

Das, S., 92
dengue virus, 8, 75, 83, 85

INDEX

Desmodium incanum, 40–41, 41f
diabetes, 7–8, 19, 24, 30–34, 98, 133, 140
diseases
  communicable, 5, 50-88, 130–32, 135, 159
  non-communicable, 4–8, 14, 23–24, 26–49, 130–32, 135, 139, 161
District of Columbia, 149
diverticulitis, 91–93
Dog Dumpling, 67–68, 67f
dogs, 48, 70
Dominica, 150
Drug Services Act, 19
drugs, 8–9, 19–20, 29, 51, 137–42, 159, 161-62
  compounds in, 9, 128, 145, 147
development of, 143, 146–48
  interactions with herbal medicines, 139-42, 157
  regulation of, 148, 150, 154
  safety of, 137, 143
Duppy Basil, 79, 79f
Duppy Needles, 30–31, 37, 52–53, 71, 127, 132
  photographs of, 31f, 37f, 53f, 71f

East Indians, 13, 149
Echinacea, 141
Eclipta prostrata, 72, 72f
education, 4, 18, 20, 154–55
Elder Bush, 31, 31f, 133
English language, 8
English Plantain, 45, 45f
English Potato, 61, 61f
epilepsy, 19, 152

Escherichia coli (E coli), 50–51, 53–54, 56, 58–59, 61–62, 64, 67–68
ethnopharmacology, 9, 16, 24, 130–31, 157, 160
Eupatorium odoratum, 72–73, 73f
Eurocentrism, 15, 17, 20–21
Europe, 10, 13–14, 134, 148–49
European Union, 154
Europeans, 10–14, 20, 127
  in Barbados, 1, 3, 5, 9, 21

Fennel, 95, 95f
Feverfew, 135
Ficus citrifolia, 1
fish, 22, 55
flavonoids, 128, 129f3.1, 130, 133, 151
  plant sources of, 27, 29–30, 32–35, 37–41, 46, 49–50, 52, 54, 56, 61–62, 67, 70–78, 80, 82–84, 88, 94, 96–97
Foeniculum vulgare, 95, 95f
folk medicine, 11, 138. *See also* traditional medicine
folklore, 127, 135, 160
Forbidden Fruit, 67–68, 67f
fossils, 126
French Cotton, 29, 29f, 86, 86f
fungal infections, 24, 85–88, 132
fungi, 24, 85–88, 126, 132, 145–46

Garlic, 13, 50–51, 50f, 94, 94f, 127, 140 41
Georgia (country), 149
Geranium, Wild or Seaside, 37, 37f, 71, 71f

INDEX

Ginger, 13, 69, 93, 100, 127, 130, 140–41, 148
  photographs of, 69f, 93f, 100f
Ginkgo biloba, 141
Ginseng, 13
Grapefruit, 140–41
Greater Antilles, 1
Guam, 149
Guava, 66, 66f
Guilandina bonduc, 74, 74f
Guyana, 3, 149, 157

Health and Wellness, Ministry of, 150
health and wellness sector, 157–58
health insurance, 19
Health Services Act, 19
Hedyotis verticillata, 82, 82f
Heliotropium angiospermum, 54, 54f
Heliotropium indicum, 54-55, 54f
hemp, 149, 154
Hepatitis B, 132
Hepatitis C, 77, 80
herbal remedies, 10, 13, 16–21, 25, 139–40, 142, 156, 159–60
  safety of, 17–18, 25, 136, 138, 156
  See also plants, medicinal use of
Herringbone, 77, 77f
Hinduism, 4, 22
Hippeastrum fosteri, 51
Hippeastrum puniceum, 51, 51f
Hog/Gully Plum, 26, 26f
Horehound, 64, 64f
Horsenicker, 74, 74f

Hot Bush, 78-79, 79f
Hug-Me-Close, 69-70, 69f
human immunodeficiency virus (HIV), 8, 72–73, 76–77, 80, 82–84, 152
Hymenaea courbaril, 78, 78f, 88, 88f, 132
Hymenocallis caribaea, 51, 51f
hypertension, 7, 19, 24, 34–49, 133, 140

India, 3
  traditional medicine of, 11, 13–14
Indian hemp, 149
Indian Root, 85–86, 86f
infectious diseases. *See* communicable diseases
influenza, 6, 8, 24, 69–73, 75, 80–82, 84–85
International Code of Nomenclature for Algae, Fungi and Plants, 126
Islam, 4, 22

Jack-in-the-Bush, 72–73, 73f
Jamaica, 3, 16, 20, 22, 149-50, 157
Jatropha curcas, 57, 57f, 86–87, 87f, 132
Judaism, 4, 22
Justicia pectoralis, 34, 35f
Justicia secunda, 35, 35f, 94, 94f

Kalanchoe pinnata, 56, 56f, 63–64, 64f, 75, 75f
Kharya, M.D., 92

INDEX

labour, 3, 12–15, 18
   indentured, 3, 11–15, 127
Lad Love, 53, 53*f*
Lantana camara, 48, 84–85, 85*f*
Lantana involucrata, 48, 48*f*
Laportea aestuans, 47, 47*f*
Latin America, 5
Latin language, 126
Lemon, 34, 34*f*
Lemongrass, 66–67, 81, 91, 99, 127, 148
   photographs of, 67*f*, 81*f*, 91*f*, 99*f*
Leonotis nepetifolia, 78–79, 79*f*
Lesser Antilles, 1
Licorice Weed, 46, 46*f*, 62, 62*f*, 83–84, 84*f*
Lilies
   Barbados/Easter, 51, 51*f*
   Spider, 51, 51*f*
Lion Head, 78–79, 79*f*
Lizard Food, 32, 39, 76, 96–97, 130
   photographs of, 32*f*, 39*f*, 76*f*, 97*f*
Lockhart, Albert, 152
Locust Tree, 78, 78*f*, 88, 88*f*, 132

Madagascar Periwinkle, 27, 27*f*, 36, 36*f*, 134–35, 148
Mahoe, 41–42, 42*f*, 80, 80*f*
Malachra alceifolia, 79–80, 79*f*
malaria, 5–6, 8, 128
Man Piabba, 78–79, 79*f*
marijuana. See *Cannabis sativa*
Marrubium vulgare, 64, 64*f*
Mauby bark, 141
medicinal plants. See plants, medicinal use of
Mentha x piperita, 97, 97*f*
Methodism, 3, 21

mice, 26, 30, 34, 99–100
Middle East, 3
Milk Weed, 57–58, 58*f*, 87, 87*f*
Miraculous Vine, 32, 39, 76, 96–97, 130
   photographs of, 32*f*, 39*f*, 76*f*, 97*f*
Momordica charantia, 32, 39, 76, 96–97, 130
   photographs of, 32*f*, 39*f*, 76*f*, 97*f*
Monkey Dumpling, 67–68, 67*f*
Monkey Fat Pork, 57, 57*f*, 86–87, 87*f*, 132
Monkey Needles, 30–31, 37, 52–53, 71, 127, 132
   photographs of, 31*f*, 37*f*, 53*f*, 71*f*
Monkey Spoon, 77, 77*f*
Moravian Church, 16
Morinda citrifolia, 67–68, 67*f*
Moringa oleifera, 33–34, 34*f*, 43, 43*f*, 65, 65*f*, 98, 98*f*
Mosquito Bush, 79, 79*f*
Myristica fragrans, 14, 90–91, 90*f*

Nagoya Protocol, 135
Neem, 33, 42, 59, 64–65, 90, 98
   photographs of, 33*f*, 42*f*, 59*f*, 65*f*, 90*f*, 98*f*
Nettle, 47, 47*f*
Nigeria, 7
non-communicable diseases, 4–8, 14, 23–24, 26–49, 130–32, 135, 139, 161
Noni, 67–68, 67*f*
North America, 3, 20, 149
Nutmeg, 14, 90–91, 90*f*
nutraceuticals, 136, 158, 161
nutrition, 5–6, 24, 161

INDEX

Obeah, 15
Ocimum campechianum, 79, 79*f*
olive oil, 50
Orisha, 21

Papaya, 27, 38, 55, 75, 90, 141
   photographs of, 27*f*, 55*f*, 75*f*, 90*f*
Parsley, 36, 36*f*, 95–96, 95*f*
Parthenium hysterophorus, 73, 73*f*, 135
Passiflora laurifolia, 44–45, 45*f*
Pear, 41, 41*f*, 92, 97–98, 97*f*
"Pen Tsao" (ancient Chinese text), 13
Pentecostalism, 3, 21
Peperomia pellucida, 28, 28*f*, 45, 45*f*, 133–34
Pepper, 14
  black, 49
  Cayenne, 68, 68*f*, 92, 92*f*
Peppermint, 97, 97*f*
Persea americana, 41, 92, 97–98
Peter, Sonia, 16
Petroselinum crispum, 36, 36*f*, 95–96, 95*f*
pharmaceuticals. *See* drugs
pharmacognosy, 9, 143, 161
pharmacokinetic antagonism, 161
phenylpropanoids, 41, 77, 85, 128, 129*f*3.1
photosynthesis, 126
Phyllanthus amarus, 27–28, 39–40, 77, 127, 132, 134
   photographs of, 28*f*, 40*f*, 77*f*
Phyllanthus epiphyllanthus, 77, 77*f*
Phyllanthus niruri, 33, 33*f*, 40, 40*f*, 127, 133

Physalis angulata, 28–29, 29*f*, 47, 47*f*, 134
Physic Nut, 57, 57*f*, 86–87, 87*f*, 132
phytochemistry, 10, 23–24, 128–42, 129*f*3.1, 151, 156–57, 161
   pharmacology and, 143–47
Pimenta racemosa, 44, 59–60, 65–66, 91, 99, 130, 148
   photographs of, 44*f*, 59*f*, 66*f*, 91*f*, 99*f*
Pineapple, 12
Plantago major, 45–46, 45*f*
plants
  biodiversity of, 8–9, 22, 127–29, 148
  Christianity and, 21–22
  drugs derived from, 143–46, 156
  medicinal use of, 8–21, 23–25, 130–43, 148, 151, 156–58
  nomenclature of, 24, 126–27
Pluchea carolinensis, 73, 74*f*, 132
Pluchea indica, 73
pollination, 11, 128
polyketides, 128, 129*f*3.1
polypharmacy, 139, 157, 161
Pop-a-gun, 32, 32*f*, 38, 38*f*
Porter Bush, 49, 49*f*, 74, 74*f*, 134
Portugal, 1
Portulaca oleracea, 30, 30*f*
Priva lappulacea, 85, 85*f*
Protestantism, 20
protists, 126
Psidium guajava, 66, 66*f*
Puerto Rico, 149
Pumpkin, 32, 39, 76, 96–97, 130
   photographs of, 32*f*, 39*f*, 76*f*, 97*f*

INDEX

Pussley, 30, 30f
Psychotria nervosa, 82, 82f
Psychotria tenuifolia, 60–61, 61f
Psychotria serpens, 82

Queen Elizabeth Hospital, 19

rabbits, 35, 91
racism, 18
Rastafari, 4, 22, 151
rats, 29, 31, 33, 36–37, 39–43, 45, 47, 49, 89, 92, 94, 133–34
Red Head, 85–86, 86f
religion, 3–4, 10, 15, 21–22
Ricinus communis, 58–59, 58f, 61
ringworm, 85–88

Sage, 48, 84–85, 85f
Seaside, 76, 76f
 Wild/Rock, 48, 48f
Santeria, 15, 21
Scoparia dulcis, 46, 46f, 62, 62f, 83–84, 84f
Seabush, 72, 72f
Seed-under-Leaf, 27–28, 33, 39–40, 77, 127, 132–34
 photographs of, 28f, 33f, 40f, 77f
Senna alata, 88, 88f
Senna occidentalis, 78, 78f
Seventh Day Adventists, 3, 21
Shango, 15
Shine Bush, 28, 28f, 45, 45f, 13334
Sida acuta, 42, 42f
Sida rhombifolia, 80, 80f
slavery, 1, 3, 5, 12–15, 17–18, 20
Snowberry, 60, 60f
Solanum tuberosum, 61, 61f

Soldier Bush, 55, 55f
solvent extracts, 42, 59, 144
Soursop, 26, 31, 35–36, 89, 94–95, 130
 photographs of, 26f, 36f, 89f, 95f
South Africa, 149
Spanish Needles, 30–31, 37, 52–53, 71, 127, 132
 photographs of, 31f, 37f, 53f, 71f
Spermacoce assurgens, 46, 46f
Spermacoce verticillata, 83, 83f
Sphagneticola trilobata, 53, 53f
Spinach, 50, 50f
Spirit Weed, 48, 48f
Spiritual Baptists, 15, 21
Spondias mombin, 26, 26f
St. John, Barbados, 130
St. John's Bush, 82, 82f
St. Kitts and Nevis, 150
St. Vincent and the Grenadines, 150
Stachytarpheta jamaicensis, 84, 84f
Staphylococcus aureus, 50–51, 53–54, 56–62, 64–69
Stinking Bush, 78, 78f
Stinking Toe Tree, 78, 78f, 88, 88f, 132
Sumeria, 10
Sweet Broom, 46, 46f, 62, 62f, 83–84, 84f
Sweetheart Bush, 40–41, 41f
Synedrella nodiflora, 49, 49f, 74, 74f, 134
synergism, 162

INDEX

Tanacetum parthenium, 135
tannins, 27, 30–31, 33, 35, 37, 39–41, 44, 47, 52, 56–57, 59, 62–64, 66, 71–72, 74, 77–78, 80, 83–86, 88–91, 95–96, 99
taxonomy, 8–9, 23–24, 126–28, 140
teas, 16–17, 26, 48, 63, 76, 82, 128, 136–37, 162
Tecoma stans, 31, 31f, 133
Terminalia catappa, 38–39, 39f
terpenoids, 10, 128, 129f3.1, 132
  plant sources of, 26, 30–34, 38–42, 44, 46, 48–52, 54–56, 59–63, 65–66, 70, 73–74, 76–78, 82–85, 91–92, 95, 97, 99
Thespesia populnea, 41–42, 42f, 80, 80f
Tim-Tom bush, 60, 60f
tourism, 3, 155
Tournefortia volubilis, 55, 55f
traditional medicine, 10–16, 18–21, 131, 137–39, 148, 156
  plants used in, 8, 23, 25, 132, 135
TRAMIL – Program of Applied Research to Popular Medicine in the Caribbean, 9, 157
trees, 21–22
Trinidad and Tobago, 3, 16, 20, 149–50, 157
Trumpet Tree, 32, 32f, 38, 38f
tuberculosis, 6, 8, 59, 65
Turmeric, 49, 62–63, 68–69, 92–93, 100, 141
  photographs of, 49f, 63f, 68f, 93f, 100f

United Nations, 4–5, 129, 149–50, 154
United States, 7, 149, 154–55
United States Food and Drug Administration (USFDA), 36, 134, 147, 151–52
Urena lobata, 81, 81f
Uruguay, 149
US Virgin Islands, 150

Vaccinium myrtillus, 56–57, 57f
vaccines, 7, 131, 148
Velvet Burr, 85, 85f
Vervain, 84, 84f
viruses, 24, 69–85
Vodou, 15, 21
Vujicic, Tatijana, 16

Water Lemon, 44–45, 45f
Wedelia, 53, 53f
West Africa, 5, 7, 11–12, 14, 127, 149
West Indian Federation, 1, 3
West Indian Tea, 61–62, 62f, 83, 83f
West Indies, 1, 149
West Indies, University of the, 24, 152
West, Manley, 152
Whitehead Bush, 73, 73f, 135
Wild Ageratum, 52, 52f, 70, 70f
Wild Clary, 54–55, 54f
Wild Coffee, 60–61, 61f
Wild Garlic, 51, 51f
Wild Okra, 79–80, 79f
Wild Olive, 43–44, 44f
Wild Pine, 67–68, 67f

Wonder of the World, 56, 56f, 63–64, 64f, 75, 75f
World Health Organization (WHO), 5, 16, 136

Yasir, M., 92
yeast, 65, 95
Yellow Foxglove, 141–42

Zingiber officinale, 13, 69, 93, 100, 127, 130, 140–41, 148
   photographs of, 69f, 93f, 100f

www.ingramcontent.com/pod-product-compliance
Lightning Source LLC
Chambersburg PA
CBHW040758120426
42983CB00044B/782